BEC | Contributors

Editors

Teri Reynolds, Nikki Roddie, Andi Tenner, Heike Geduld.

Other contributors of written material

Kalie Dove-Maguire, Vijay Kannan, Sean Kivlehan, Nelson Olim, Max Ritzenberg, Stas Salerno Amato, Morgan Broccoli, Farrah Kashfipour, Harald Veen, Lee Wallis

Peer reviewers

Annet Alenyo, John Brown, Emilie Calvello, Brendan Carr, Keegan Checkett, Matthew Cooke, Megan Cox, Anne Creaton, Rochelle Dicker, Shaheem De Vries, Stephen Dunlop, Rajith Ellawala, George Etoundi, Sabariah Faizah, Scott Fruhan, Nicolaus Glomb, Renee Hsia, Christina Huwer, Muhumpu Kafwamfwa, Joseph Kalanzi, Gamal Khalifa, Olive Kobusingye, Clifford Mann, Edgardo Menendez, Juma Mfinanga, Nee-Kofi Mould-Millman, Hani Mowafi, Andrew Muck, Brittany Murray, Marcos Musafir, Theresa Olasveengen, Gerard O'Reilly, Tom Potokar, Junaid Razzak, Anthony Redmond, Andres Rubiano, Kelly Schmiedeknecht, Chris Stein, Janis Tupesis, Vikas Kapil, and Benjamin Wachira.

The following members of the International Liaison Committee on Resuscitation (ILCOR) Pediatric Task Force provided essential peer review on relevant sections: Ng Kee Chong, Allan de Caen, Ian Maconochie, and Remigio Véiz.

The following members of the International Federation for Emergency Medicine executive committee provided essential peer review: Peter Cameron, James Ducharme, Jim Holliman, Bob Schafermeyer, and Andrew Singer.

Focus groups and pilots

We thank the nurses and doctors of Muhimbili National Hospital in Dar es Salaam, United Republic of Tanzania, for their invaluable input during early focus groups: Ally M. Akrabi, Prosper J. Bashaka, Avelina N. Ijumba, Jennifer Jamieson, Khadija H. Juma, Bernard Kepha, Said Kilindimo, Josephine Lazaro, Wendy Lukwambe, Peter S. Mabula, Deogratius Mally, Nyakanda Marwa, Juma Mbugi, Felix D. Mlay, Victoria Mlele, Brittany Murray, Kissa Mwampagama, Meera Nariadhara, Catherine R. Shari, Patrick J. Shao, Shahzmah Suleman, Renatus Tarimo, Tito William.

We are grateful to the African Federation for Emergency Medicine for overall coordination of pilots conducted in 2015–2017.

Uganda course pilots were led by Joseph Kalanzi, and course facilitators included Aliga Cliff Asher, Charmaine Cunningham, Heike Geduld, Nemganga Kizega, Namaganda Lukia, Grace Magambo, Alex Makupe, Juma Mbugi, Josephine Nabulime, Annet Alenyo Ngabirano, Muzaza Nthele. Participants: Halima Adam, Douglas Akibua, Muhwezi Amos, Beatrice Babirye, Andrew Balinda, Evans Bonabana, Kamara Francis, Alele Franco, Muduwa Grace, Jagwe Hakim, Henry

Kagaba, Shadia Kaggwa, Andrew Kagwa, Peter Kavuma, Winnie Kibirige, Bazibu Musa Kireka, Brian Kisembo, Nakiyemba Margaret, Edward Mugisha, Linda Nalugya, Gertrude Namidembe, Joanita Namuddu, Denis Onyang, and Emma Tukehayo.

United Republic of Tanzania course pilots were led by Hendry Sawe, and course facilitators included Charmaine Cunningham, Jimmy Ernest, Upendo George, Nemganga Kizega, Deogratius Mally, Juma Mbugi, Juma Mfinanga, Felix Mlay, Brittany L Murray, Suzanna Ngalla, and Nikki Roddie. Participants: Ntuli Abraham, Thomas Bwire, Hamza Haji, Agripina Hugho, Stella Ibrahim, Philomena Jumanne, Teonila Kamba, Neema Kayembe, Sikudhani Khamsini, Clemence Luambono, Raymond Makona, Rosemary Marishay, Rashidi Matitu, Vicent Mboya, Erick Mhaiki, Rashid Mhina, Asha Mkwachu, Frank Mlaguzi, Leonidas Mutakosa, Piensia Nanyimbula, Kiohombo Phim, Mary Shauritanga, and Ndamba Sigonda.

Zambia course pilots were led by Muhumpu Kafwamfwa, and course facilitators included: Namasiku Chime, Chipoya Chipoya, Ngandu Hassan, Mwandameda Kabuku, Irene Lufunda, Alex Makupe, and Mzaza Nthele. Participants: Gloria Chambeshi, Maureen Chikwa, Azelina Chulu, Mwanza Jackson, Usaliwa Jere, Tina Malunga, Pidini Mary, Mable Nakazwe Mulenga, Joy Judy Mweshi, Chicco Siame, Ivan Sinaulieni, and Franko Zulu.

We wish to thank Morgan Broccoli, Simon Charwey, Catherine Haeffele, Farrah Kashfipour for input on visual design and illustration, and Tein Jung for the original illustrations throughout.

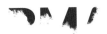

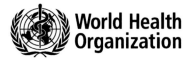World Health Organization

ICRC

BASIC EMERGENCY CARE

APPROACH TO THE ACUTELY ILL AND INJURED

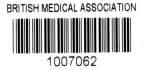

Basic emergency care: approach to the acutely ill and injured

ISBN (WHO) 978–92–4-151308–1
ISBN (ICRC) 978–2-940396–58–0

Design by Inís Communication – www.iniscommunication.com

Contents

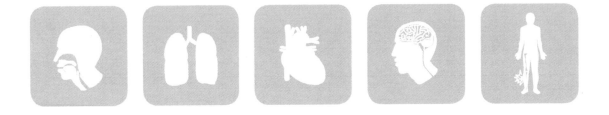

INTRODUCTION

Overview

Health emergencies happen every day, everywhere. They affect adults and children and include injuries and infections, heart attacks and strokes, acute complications of pregnancy and of chronic disease. While specialised care may never be available at all times in all places, a systematic approach to emergency conditions saves lives. The Disease Control Priorities Project estimates that nearly half of deaths and a third of disabilities in low- and middle-income countries result from conditions that could be addressed by emergency care.

The World Health Organization (WHO), in collaboration with the International Committee of the Red Cross (ICRC) and the International Federation for Emergency Medicine (IFEM), has developed the Basic Emergency Care (BEC) course for frontline providers who manage acute life-threatening conditions with limited resources. These may include students, nurses, pre-hospital technicians, clinical officers and doctors who are working in field (pre-hospital) or hospital settings.

Emergency care providers must respond to 'undifferentiated' patients, those with acute symptoms for which the cause may not be known. This course introduces a systematic approach to managing acute, potentially life-threatening conditions even before a diagnosis is known.

BEC is based on the clinical recommendations of the WHO *IMAI District Clinician Manual*, WHO *Pocket Book of Hospital Care for Children*, WHO *Emergency Triage Assessment and Treatment (ETAT)* and WHO *Integrated Management of Pregnancy and Childbirth*. It includes modules on: the ABCDE and SAMPLE history approach, trauma, difficulty in breathing, shock, and altered mental status. The practical skills section covers the essential time-sensitive interventions for these key acute presentations.

The WHO BEC package consists of:

- *Participant workbook*: the main reference source for participants, this interactive workbook provides all the necessary course content, and includes an in-depth guide to essential skills, a glossary of terms, review questions and case scenarios.

- *Quick cards*: these simple reference cards organize key assessment and management points for use in clinical settings beyond the course. These are found at the end of each module and together at the end of the workbook.

- *Facilitator guide:* this is an annotated version of the BEC workbook intended for facilitators. Challenging concepts are highlighted, and notes on teaching strategy and lecture preparation provided on each page. This volume also includes a Coordinator section with information on course planning and logistics, and offers guidance for selecting and training facilitators.

- *Presentation slide sets:* these cover all course modules and are provided to support course delivery.

INTRO

ABCDE

TRAUMA

BREATHING

SHOCK

AMS

SKILLS

GLOSSARY

REFS & QUICK CARDS

The BEC course may be implemented in many different ways to meet local needs, but a recommended 5-day schedule is described in detail in the Coordinator section of the Facilitator guide. The BEC content might also be spread across a few weeks as a module in undergraduate nursing or medical curricula. The BEC package is designed to support the efforts of governments, educational institutions, professional societies and others to train emergency care providers acting within their designated scope of practice. WHO does not certify or accredit courses, instructors or providers.

Scope of the course

Key acute presentations

These modules teach a practical and systematic approach to four acute and potentially life-threatening presentations:

- Trauma
- Difficulty in breathing
- Shock
- Altered mental status

Most life-threatening conditions, whether the original cause was medical or surgical, infection or injury, will present with one of these. In some cases the diagnosis may be known, while in others, intervention may be required before a diagnosis can be made, perhaps because of limited diagnostic resources, but often because of the acuity of the condition. These modules introduce a systematic approach to assessment and management that can be used whether or not a diagnosis has been made.

Frontline health-care providers will face many more presentations than are covered in this course. This material is not meant to cover every acute condition, but to help providers address time-sensitive conditions where early intervention has the potential to save lives. The course is designed to lay a foundation for broader emergency assessment and management. Many participants may already, or will later, be trained to provide care beyond what is described here. Recommendations for handover to an "advanced provider" are meant to signal the need for care beyond the scope of this course. In some cases, participants themselves may already be trained to provide this additional care.

Other emergency presentations

There are other complaints that may represent a life-threatening condition requiring emergency care even before it progresses to any of the key acute presentations listed above. These include:

- chest discomfort;
- poisoning/ingestion/exposure;
- envenomation (bites/stings);
- any severe pain from an unclear source;

- contractions, pain or bleeding in late pregnancy.

These complaints may represent the early stage of a critical illness requiring rapid intervention even when the person appears relatively well. The complete assessment and management of these conditions is beyond the scope of this course, but they should always trigger transport to, or consultation with, an advanced provider.

In addition, there are certain infectious exposures that require time-sensitive prophylaxis (preventive treatment) whose effectiveness may be reduced by delays. These include:

- needle stick injury in a health care worker;
- unprotected sexual encounter, including in the context of assault;
- exposure to the saliva of an animal with suspected rabies.

These exposures should be evaluated as soon as possible at a center capable of providing timely prophylaxis.

Special considerations for fever

Fever is a very common complaint and may be a sign of a life-threatening condition, or simply a sign of a mild condition that will resolve itself. Because fever does not reliably indicate an emergency condition, it is not addressed in a separate module here, but is covered in each of the core modules. When associated with abnormal ABCDE findings (see "Approach to the emergency patient" section), or any of the acute presentations above (trauma, difficulty in breathing, shock, altered mental status), fever can be an important clue to severe illness and should be taken very seriously. There are many more causes of fever than can be covered in this basic course, but most causes of fever requiring emergency treatment are associated with one of the four key acute presentations.

There is no single approach to fever that is right for all emergencies, but there are some general principles that can help in the assessment and management of emergency patients.

- Always consider infection in a person with fever (e.g. malaria, meningitis, pneumonia).
- Never use the absence of fever to rule out infection. People with overwhelming infection or immune system problems may not be able to produce a fever and may have a normal or low body temperature.
- Fever with abnormal vital signs and/or any of the four key acute conditions listed above will likely require early antibiotic (and/or anti-malarial) treatment.
- Always consider whether local screening protocols for infectious disease outbreaks (e.g. for haemorrhagic fevers) require further action (e.g. special reporting or management) in a person with fever.

Obstetric delivery and neonatal resuscitation

Management of obstetric delivery and neonatal resuscitation are critical topics covered elsewhere in existing WHO materials and are not covered in this course. See the WHO Maternal, Newborn, Child and Adolescent Health department website (http://www.who.int/maternal_child_adolescent/documents/en/) for training materials on these topics.

Expected participant background knowledge

This course assumes a basic knowledge in the following areas:

- Use of personal protective equipment
- Basic human anatomy
- Basic history taking
- Basic physical examination skills, including taking vital signs, chest auscultation and abdominal assessment
- Use of a glucometer
- Set up of an intravenous (IV) infusion
- Safe intramuscular injection
- Cardiopulmonary resuscitation (CPR)

Cardiopulmonary resuscitation (CPR)

The decision about whether or not CPR is appropriate for a specific patient depends on many factors, including understanding of the cause of the condition, knowledge of available resources, and awareness of relevant institutional protocols and practices. There are many situations where it may be appropriate to initiate and then terminate CPR after a certain interval, and others where it may not be appropriate to initiate CPR. While this course addresses several aspects of resuscitation, it does not cover general CPR protocols, as they may vary greatly by setting. Course facilitators should direct participants to the appropriate source for relevant CPR protocols.

Medication

The medications discussed in this course are widely available and appropriate for use by the frontline providers for whom the course is designed. They can be used in pre-hospital or facility-based settings and are important early treatments for emergency conditions. The included medications provide a foundation for initial emergency care, but almost every condition discussed in this workbook will require treatments beyond those listed. Many important emergency treatments used by advanced providers are not included in this course.

Handover/transfer

This course is designed to help providers identify and provide initial management for acute, life-threatening conditions. Most acutely ill patients will require care beyond this initial stage. This may be ongoing care delivered by the same provider, but more often will require handover to a more advanced provider or facility. This process of deciding the appropriate disposition – or next step of care – for the acutely ill patient is a vital part of emergency care. Choosing an appropriate disposition involves assessing severity; estimating how rapidly the condition may progress; considering whether transfer for a specific intervention (e.g. surgery, blood transfusion) is needed; and identifying any specific risks based on a suspected or known diagnosis (e.g. risk of recurrent seizure/convulsion, or worsening airway blockage). The special disposition considerations for each key acute presentation and its associated diagnoses are covered in the modules.

Planning for handover/transfer requires communicating essential information with the receiving facility, creating a transport plan, and ensuring availability of the necessary supplies to protect providers and care for patients. These components will be covered in detail in "Transfer and handover" in the Skills section.

Triage

Triage is the systematic process of classifying patients by acuity to ensure the best match between available resources and user needs. Triage is an essential component of emergency care during routine and surge conditions, and is a higher-level process applied to all patients, allowing assessment of the individual patient in context. As such, it is not addressed in this course, but is often taught at the same time. WHO and ICRC, in collaboration with Médecins Sans Frontières (MSF) and the South African Triage Score (SATS) team, have developed a set of integrated triage tools and an associated open-access training module. Contact **emergencycare@who.int** to request these materials.

Approach to the emergency patient

The BEC course is intended for a wide range of frontline providers and offers a basic approach for life-threatening presentations. Emergency conditions often require urgent intervention long before a diagnosis is established, and a presentation-based approach is essential to managing patients effectively. The modules in this course teach the elements of a general approach that can be used for any emergency patient. *Aaron*

The ABCDE approach allows rapid assessment and intervention for life threats using the following categories:

A: **AIRWAY**

B: **BREATHING**

C: **CIRCULATION**

D: **DISABILITY**

E: **EXPOSURE**

Essential ABCDE considerations are listed in the modules for each of the four key presentations.

The SAMPLE history is a method of rapidly gathering the history critical to the management of the acutely ill patient. The SAMPLE history categories are:

S: **SIGNS AND SYMPTOMS**

A: **ALLERGIES**

M: **MEDICATIONS**

P: **PAST MEDICAL HISTORY**

L: **LAST ORAL INTAKE**

E: **EVENTS SURROUNDING ILLNESS**

Essential SAMPLE questions are listed in the modules for each of the four key presentations.

The secondary survey is a complete physical examination based on the specific condition. The essential relevant components of the secondary survey are listed in the modules for each of the four key presentations. Further details are covered in the Skills section.

How to use this Participant Workbook

This Participant Workbook is linked with the WHO BEC course presentations and is designed to help participants prepare for each lesson to maximize learning. Each module provides reading material and exercises to complete **before** the lesson. Participants should not worry if there are elements they do not fully understand while reading alone, as all workbook content will be reviewed during the lessons.

Before each lesson, participants should:

- write out the definitions for the **Key terms** of the relevant module by copying from the **Glossary** in the back of the workbook;
- complete all workbook review questions in the relevant modules.

The multiple choice questions and case scenarios at the end of each module will be covered in the small group sessions during the course, but participants should read through them before the session.

On completion of the course, participants can use this book for reference. Accompanying the book are *reference quick cards.* These cards provide a summary of the essential points from the course and are designed to be carried in the clinical setting to guide day-to-day practice.

Module format

This course includes one module on the general approach to all emergency patients (ABCDE and SAMPLE); one module on the approach to injured patients (trauma); three modules on other specific clinical presentations (difficulty in breathing, shock, and altered mental status); a skills section; and a Glossary.

The modules include the following sections:

Objectives: A list of things participants should be able to do by the end of the course.

Essential skills: A list of skills relevant to the module (and later taught in the Skills section).

Key terms: Important words and phrases needed to understand the module. All definitions can be found in the Glossary and should be written in the space provided prior to the lecture.

Overview: A brief introduction to the clinical presentation being discussed in the module.

Goals of initial assessment: The main purpose of the assessment of the clinical presentation.

Goals of acute management: The desired result of the management of the clinical condition.

ABCDE key elements: ABCDE findings and interventions related to the specific clinical condition addressed in the module.

Key history findings (ASK): Specific SAMPLE history elements related to the clinical presentation that are critical for management.

PARTICIPANT WORKBOOK

INTRO

ABCDE

TRAUMA

BREATHING

SHOCK

AMS

SKILLS

GLOSSARY

REFS & QUICK CARDS

Secondary survey findings (CHECK, including Look, Listen and Feel): Relevant secondary examination findings to check for in the clinical presentation the module addresses.

Possible causes: Specific diseases, injuries, or illnesses that can cause the condition presented in the module (along with their specific signs and symptoms).

Management (DO): These sections describe management of specific conditions. Note that the *ABCDE* and *Trauma* modules have much longer lists of possible emergency conditions, and the *Possible causes* and *Management* sections are presented in tables. The *Trauma* module has a separate table for Primary Survey conditions.

Special considerations in children: Important differences in the signs and symptoms and management needs of children.

Disposition considerations: Specific things to consider when transferring or handing over patients.

Facilitator-led case scenarios: These scenarios test participants' ability to use what they have learned to manage a patient. These scenarios will be led by the instructor.

Multiple choice questions (MCQ): There are five multiple choice questions to test your knowledge at the end of each module in preparation for the final written exam.

Participant requirements

Participants should confirm course requirements with their facilitator. When implemented in full, the Basic Emergency Care course requires completion of **ALL** components listed below.

Pre-test. Before receiving the Basic Emergency Care course workbook, participants should have completed this brief confidential test, which helps facilitators understand their current knowledge level.

Attendance report. Participants must sign in for both the morning and afternoon sessions each day. **Participants must attend all sessions to pass the course.**

Workbook completion. As described above, **participants should complete all *key terms* and *workbook questions*** in the relevant module prior to each lesson. All key terms must be defined, and all workbook questions answered for the workbook to be considered completed. The workbooks will be reviewed each day by facilitators. **Participants must complete the workbook to pass the course.**

Skill stations. During the skills day, facilitators will demonstrate skills at a practical station. Participants will have an opportunity to practise the skill at each station several times. Participants may practise a skill as many times as needed within the allotted station time. During practice, participants may use the workbook and skill checklist for reference, and may ask questions as needed of facilitators. During assessment, no reference materials will be allowed, so participants should also practise without references, and have another participant observe for any missed steps. Participants will have plenty of time to practise and feel confident with the skills prior to assessment, and when ready, should request that an instructor assess them performing the skill. All steps in the skill checklist must be performed to pass the assessment. **Participants must pass the skill station assessments to pass the course.**

Case scenarios. **All participants must successfully lead and manage a case scenario to pass the course.** These scenarios give participants an opportunity to practise an integrated approach to management in small groups of 3–4 participants. Facilitators will discuss with the group how to approach the case scenarios using the ABCDE approach. In the later modules, each participant will be assessed on the ability to lead and manage a case scenario. Leading a case scenario includes identifying critical aspects of assessment and management, as well as presenting a handover summary (see the Handover section in Skills). Facilitators will complete the checklist below to assess the participant leading the case. Participants who are unsuccessful in identifying and managing the critical conditions in the scenario will be given a second case in the same or a subsequent session. Assessments are based on a standardized guide and reported on the form below.

Case scenario assessment	Not identified	Identified some	Identified all
Critical airway interventions			
Critical breathing interventions			
Critical circulation interventions			
Critical disability interventions			
Critical exposure interventions			
Critical medications (if needed)			
Gave appropriate brief handover summary	Yes	No	
Participant performed all essential components	Yes	No	

Comments (including notation of any missed elements):

Written final exam

To qualify to sit the final examination participants must:

- complete the pre-test;
- complete the key terms and workbook questions;
- attend all course sessions;
- lead a case scenario;
- pass all skill stations as examined by an instructor.

The final examination will include multiple choice questions.

Participants must score at least 75% to pass.

Your input will help improve future training courses. Please send any comments, corrections or questions to *emergencycare@who.int*. We encourage all participants and facilitators to fill out a short pre- and post-course survey at *www.who.int/emergencycare*.

The ABCDE and SAMPLE history approach

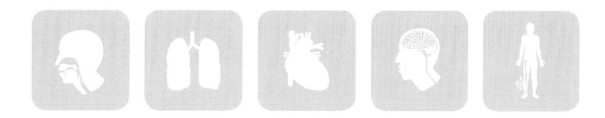

Notes

Module 1: The ABCDE and SAMPLE history approach

OBJECTIVES

On completing this module you should be able to:

1. list the hazards that must be considered when approaching an ill or injured person;

2. list the elements to approaching an ill or injured person safely;

3. list the components of the systematic ABCDE approach to emergency patients;

4. assess an airway;

5. explain when to use airway devices;

6. explain when advanced airway management is needed;

7. assess breathing;

8. explain when to assist breathing;

9. assess fluid status (circulation);

10. provide appropriate fluid resuscitation;

11. describe the critical ABCDE actions;

12. list the elements of a SAMPLE history;

13. perform a relevant SAMPLE history.

Essential skills

• Assessing ABCDE	• Glucose administration
• Cervical spine immobilization	• Needle decompression for tension pneumothorax
• Full spine immobilization	• Three-sided dressing for chest wound
• Head-tilt and chin-lift/jaw thrust	• Intravenous (IV) line placement
• Airway suctioning	• IV fluid resuscitation
• Management of choking	• Direct pressure for haemorrhage control, including deep wound packing
• Recovery position	• Tourniquet for haemorrhage control
• Nasopharyngeal and oropharyngeal airway placement	• Pelvic binding
• Bag-valve-mask ventilation	• Wound management
• Oxygen administration	• Fracture immobilization
• Skin pinch test	• Snake bite management
• AVPU (alert, voice, pain, unresponsive) assessment	

INTRO

ABCDE

TRAUMA

BREATHING

SHOCK

AMS

SKILLS

GLOSSARY

REFS & QUICK CARDS

KEY TERMS

Write the definition using the Glossary at the back of the workbook.

ABCDE:

Accessory muscle use:

Altered mental status (AMS):

Anaphylaxis:

AVPU:

Bag-valve-mask (BVM):

Capillary refill:

Cardiopulmonary resuscitation (CPR):

Cervical spine (c-spine):

Convulsion:

Crackles (crepitations):

Crepitus:

Deep wound packing:

Defibrillator:

Diaphoresis:

Difficulty in breathing (DIB):

Disposition:

Foreign body:

GCS (Glasgow Coma Scale):

Hives:

Haematoma:

Haemorrhage:

Haemothorax:

Hyperresonance:

Hyperthermia:

Hypoglycaemia:

Hypothermia:

Hypotension:

Hypoxia:

Inhalation injury:

Intubation:

Large bore IV:

Nasal flaring:

Nasopharyngeal airway (NPA):

Needle decompression:

Oedema:

Oropharyngeal airway (OPA):

Oxygen saturation (O₂ sat):

Percussion:

_____

Perfusion:

_____

Pericardial tamponade:

_____

Personal protective equipment (PPE):

_____

Pleural effusion:

_____

Pneumothorax:

_____

Pulse oximeter:

_____

Retractions:

_____

SAMPLE history:

_____

Seizure:

_____

Shock:

_____

Stridor:

_____

Sucking chest wound:

_____

Tachypnoea:

_____

Tension pneumothorax:

_____

Wheezing:

_____

INTRO

ABCDE

TRAUMA

BREATHING

SHOCK

AMS

SKILLS

GLOSSARY

REFS & QUICK CARDS

OVERVIEW

Approaching every patient in a systematic way ensures that life-threatening conditions are recognized promptly and that the most critical interventions are done first. In a stable patient, the initial ABCDE approach may only take seconds to a few minutes. The ABCDE should be followed by a rapid history using the SAMPLE approach (Signs and Symptoms, Allergies, Medications, Past medical history, Last oral intake and Events). The SAMPLE history categories are described in general below, and essential questions for a specific presentation are listed in the relevant module. Using the standard SAMPLE and ABCDE approach together ensures that different providers can easily communicate about acutely ill patients.

> **The goal of the ABCDE approach** is to rapidly identify life-threatening conditions; ensure the airway stays open; and ensure that breathing and circulation are adequate to deliver oxygen to the body.
>
> **The goal of the SAMPLE approach** is to rapidly gather history critical to the management of the acutely ill patient.

This module will address:

- Safety considerations
- Elements of the ABCDE approach
- In-depth: acute life-threatening conditions (signs, symptoms and management)
- Paediatric considerations in the ABCDE approach
- Elements of the SAMPLE history
- Disposition considerations

SAFETY CONSIDERATIONS

A critical part of the approach to any ill or injured patient is keeping providers and others safe. An ill or injured provider will be unable to help anyone, and instead becomes an extra patient for other responders to treat. Safety consideration involves checking for:

- **scene hazards.** Is there a fire, electrical wire or chemical spill that could injure providers or bystanders? At a road traffic crash, is the scene closed to oncoming traffic? If a building has collapsed, is it safe to enter? At the scene of an explosion, always consider the possibility of further explosions. Remember that delayed building collapse may follow explosions, fires and earthquakes.

- **violence.** Is there a chance that providers may be harmed by the patient or by others? For patients who are aggressive or agitated, request help as needed from security personnel or police before beginning your assessment.

- **infectious disease risk.** Is there a possibility for disease exposure (such as flu or haemorrhagic fever)?

USE PERSONAL PROTECTIVE EQUIPMENT

You may not know the cause of illness or injury when you first approach a patient, and without appropriate personal protective equipment (PPE), may expose yourself to diseases, chemicals or poisons. You must use appropriate PPE every time you approach a patient. Always protect yourself from any exposure to bodily fluids. This will almost always require gloves and eye protection, and may require a gown and mask. Some circumstances, such as suspected or confirmed haemorrhagic fever outbreaks, require specific protective practices. Always be sure that you are up-to-date on current local recommendations.

CLEANING AND DECONTAMINATION

Infectious disease exposure is a significant risk. Use PPE and wash your hands before and after every patient contact. At the scene, hand washing may not be immediately possible; carry an alcohol gel cleanser if possible. Between patients, clean and disinfect all facility and vehicle surfaces and all reusable equipment.

Decontamination may be required after exposure to pesticides or other chemicals (dry or wet) and, depending on the chemical, may include washing or brushing to remove the substance. Not all chemicals can be safely washed away, and some must be removed in specific ways to avoid further injury. You must wear appropriate PPE for this. Refer to local decontamination protocols for people and equipment.

ASK FOR MORE HELP IF NEEDED

- If multiple people are injured or ill, call for help or send someone to call.
- If advanced care is needed, begin making arrangements as early as possible for consultations or transfers.
- Know the relevant local agencies to contact for suspected outbreaks or hazardous exposures, such as chemical spills or radiation. There is often support and guidance available for containment and decontamination.

Workbook question 1: Safety

A person walks into your health post vomiting, bleeding from the mouth, and complaining of abdominal pain.

Using the workbook section above, describe what is needed to safely approach this person:

_____

_____

_____

_____

ELEMENTS OF THE ABCDE APPROACH

The ABCDE approach

The ABCDE approach provides a framework for the systematic and organized evaluation of acutely ill patients in order to rapidly identify and intervene for life-threatening conditions:

A – Airway: check for and correct any obstruction to movement of air into the lungs

B – Breathing: ensure adequate movement of air into the lungs

C – Circulation: evaluate whether there is adequate perfusion to deliver oxygen to the tissues; check for signs of life-threatening bleeding

D – Disability: assess and protect brain and spine functions

E – Exposure: identify all injuries and any environmental threats and avoid hypothermia

This stepwise approach is designed to ensure that life-threatening conditions can be identified and treated early, in order of priority. If a problem is discovered in any of these steps, it must be addressed immediately before moving on to the next step. The ABCDE approach should be performed in the first 5 minutes and repeated whenever a patient's condition changes or worsens.

INTRO

ABCDE

TRAUMA

BREATHING

SHOCK

AMS

SKILLS

GLOSSARY

REFS & QUICK CARDS

THE ABCDE ASSESSMENT AND MANAGEMENT

> **REMEMBER...** Always check for signs of trauma in each of the ABCDE sections, and reference the trauma module as needed. [see TRAUMA]

	ASSESSMENT	IMMEDIATE MANAGEMENT

Airway	Can the patient talk normally? If YES, the airway is open.
	
	If the patient cannot talk normally:
	
	• look to see if the chest wall is moving and listen to see if there is air movement from the mouth or nose.
	• listen for abnormal sounds (such as stridor, grunting, or snoring) or a hoarse or raspy voice that indicates a partially obstructed airway.
	  – Stridor plus swelling and/or hives suggest a severe allergic reaction (anaphylaxis).
	
	• Look and listen for fluid (such as blood, vomit) in the airway.
	• Look for foreign body or abnormal swelling around the airway, and altered mental status.
	• Check if the patient is able to swallow saliva or is drooling.
		• If the patient is unconscious and not breathing normally and:
		  – NO TRAUMA: open the airway using the **head-tilt and chin-lift** manoeuvre. [See SKILLS]
		  – CONCERN FOR TRAUMA: maintain cervical spine immobilization and open the airway using the **jaw thrust** manoeuvre. [See SKILLS]
		  – Place an **oropharyngeal or nasopharyngeal airway** to maintain the airway. [See SKILLS]
		
		• If a foreign body is suspected:
		  – If the object is visible, remove it – be careful not to push the object any deeper.
		  – If the patient is able to cough or make noises, keep the patient calm and encourage coughing.
		  – If the patient is choking (unable to cough, not making sounds) use age-appropriate **chest thrusts/ abdominal thrusts/back blows**. [See SKILLS]
		  – If the patient becomes unconscious while choking, follow relevant **CPR** protocols.
		
		• If secretions or vomit are present, **suction** when available, or wipe clean. Consider placing patient in the recovery position if the rest of the ABCDE is normal and no trauma is suspected. [See SKILLS]
		
		• If the patient has swelling, hives or stridor, consider severe allergic reaction (anaphylaxis), and give **intramuscular adrenaline**. [See SKILLS]
		
		• Allow the patient to stay in a position of comfort and prepare for rapid **handover/transfer** to a centre capable of advanced airway management, if needed.

If the airway is open, move onto "Breathing".

INTRO

ABCDE

TRAUMA

BREATHING

SHOCK

AMS

SKILLS

GLOSSARY

REFS & QUICK CARDS

	ASSESSMENT	IMMEDIATE MANAGEMENT
Breathing	• Look, listen, and feel to see if the patient is breathing.	• If unconscious with abnormal breathing, start **bag-valve-mask ventilation** and follow relevant **CPR** protocols.
	• Assess if breathing is very fast, very slow, or very shallow.	• If not breathing adequately (too slow for age or too shallow), begin **bag-valve-mask ventilation with oxygen** [See SKILLS]. If oxygen not immediately available, DO NOT DELAY ventilation. Start ventilation while oxygen is being prepared. Plan for rapid handover/transfer.
	• Look for signs of increased work of breathing (such as accessory muscle use, chest indrawing/retractions, nasal flaring) or abnormal chest wall movement.	
	• Listen for abnormal breath sounds such as wheezing or crackles. [See DIFFICULTY IN BREATHING]	• If breathing fast or hypoxic, give **oxygen** [See SKILLS]
	• With severe wheezing, there may be limited/no breath sounds on examination because narrowing of the airways may be so severe that breathing cannot be heard.	• If wheezing, give **salbutamol**. [See SKILLS] Repeat salbutamol as needed.
		• If concern for severe allergic reaction (anaphylaxis), give intramuscular adrenaline. [See SKILLS]
	• Listen to see if breath sounds are equal on both sides.	• If concern for tension pneumothorax, perform needle decompression immediately and give IV fluids and oxygen. [See SKILLS] Plan for rapid handover/transfer.
	• Check for the absence of breath sounds and dull sounds with percussion on one side (large pleural effusion or haemothorax). [See SKILLS]	
	• If there are no breath sounds on one side, and hypotension, check for distended neck veins or a shifted trachea (tension pneumothorax).	• If concern for large pleural effusion or haemothorax, give oxygen and plan for rapid handover/transfer.
	• Check oxygen saturation with a pulse oximeter when available.	• *If cause unknown, remember the possibility of trauma* [See TRAUMA]

If breathing is adequate, move onto "Circulation".

	ASSESSMENT	IMMEDIATE MANAGEMENT
Circulation	• Look and feel for signs of poor perfusion (cool, moist extremities, delayed capillary refill greater than 3 seconds, low blood pressure, tachypnoea, tachycardia, absent pulses).	• For cardiopulmonary arrest, follow relevant CPR protocols.
		• If signs of poor perfusion, give IV fluids and oxygen [See SKILLS] and:
	• Look for both external AND internal bleeding, including bleeding:	– For external bleeding, apply direct pressure or use other technique to control. [See SKILLS]
	– into chest;	
	– into abdomen;	– If internal bleeding or pericardial tamponade are suspected, refer rapidly to a centre with surgical capabilities.
	– from stomach or intestine;	
	– from pelvic or femur fracture;	
	– from wounds.	*If cause unknown, remember the possibility of trauma:* Bind pelvic fractures and splint femur fractures, or any fracture with compromised blood flow. [See TRAUMA and SKILLS]
	• Look for hypotension, distended neck veins and muffled heart sounds that might indicate pericardial tamponade.	

If circulation is adequate, move onto "Disability".

	ASSESSMENT	IMMEDIATE MANAGEMENT
Disability	• Assess level of consciousness with the AVPU scale (Alert, Voice, Pain, Unresponsive) or in trauma cases, the Glasgow Coma Scale (GCS). [See SKILLS] • Always check glucose level in the confused or unconscious patient. • Check for pupil size, whether the pupils are equal, and if pupils are reactive to light. • Check movement and sensation in all four limbs. • Look for abnormal repetitive movements or shaking on one or both sides of the body (seizure/convulsion).	• If altered mental status and no evidence of trauma, place in recovery position. [See SKILLS] • If glucose low (<3.5 mmol/L) or glucose test not available and patient has altered mental status, give glucose. [See SKILLS] • For active seizures, give a benzodiazepine. [See SKILLS] • If pregnant and having seizures, give magnesium sulphate. [See SKILLS] • If pupils are small and breathing slow, consider opioid overdose and give naloxone. [See SKILLS] • If pupils are not equal, consider increased pressure on the brain and raise head of bed 30 degrees if no concern for spinal injury. Plan for rapid transfer to an advanced provider or facility with neurosurgical care. ***If cause unknown, remember possibility of trauma:*** Immobilize the cervical spine if concern for trauma. [See TRAUMA and SKILLS]
Exposure	• Examine the entire body for hidden injuries, rashes, bites or other lesions. • Rashes, such as hives, can indicate allergic reaction, and other rashes can indicate serious infection.	• If snake bite is suspected, immobilize the limb. [See SKILLS] Take a picture of the snake if possible from a distance and send with patient. Do not risk additional bites to catch/kill snake. • Remove constricting clothing and all jewelry. • Cover the patient as soon as possible to prevent hypothermia. Acutely ill patients have difficulty regulating body temperature. • Remove any wet clothes and dry patient thoroughly. • Respect the patient and protect modesty during exposure. ***If cause unknown, remember the possibility of trauma:*** Log roll if suspected spinal injury [See TRAUMA and SKILLS]

ABCDE IN DEPTH: ACUTE, LIFE-THREATENING CONDITIONS

This section takes a deeper look at conditions that must be managed during the ABCDE approach.

AIRWAY conditions

CONDITION	SIGNS AND SYMPTOMS	IN-DEPTH DESCRIPTION AND MANAGEMENT

Obstruction due to foreign body	• Visible secretions, vomit or foreign bodies in the airway
	• Abnormal sounds from the airway (such as stridor, snoring, gurgling)
	• Mental status changes leading to airway obstruction from the tongue
	• Poor chest rise
		The airway can become obstructed by secretions, vomit or foreign bodies.
		• Remove the foreign body if possible and suction fluid. Be careful not to push a foreign body further into the airway. Do not try to remove a foreign body unless clearly visible.
		• Use age-appropriate chest thrusts/abdominal thrusts/back blows if the airway is completely obstructed. [See SKILLS]
		• The tongue may obstruct the airway in patients with a decreased level of consciousness.
		  – Open the airway using a head-tilt and chin-lift manoeuvre, or use jaw thrust (if there is concern for trauma); and place an oral or nasopharyngeal airway as needed. [See SKILLS]
		  – These patients may also not be able to protect their airway and need to be watched for vomiting and aspiration.
		• Plan for rapid handover/transfer to advanced provider capable of advanced airway management if the obstruction cannot be removed.

Obstruction due to burns	• Burns to head and neck • Burned nasal hairs or soot around the nose or mouth • Abnormal sounds from the airway (such as stridor) • Change in voice • Poor chest rise	Burns can cause airway swelling due to inhalational injuries. • Give oxygen to ALL patients with suspected airway burn even if they do not show signs of hypoxia. [See SKILLS] • Open the airway using appropriate manoeuvre and place an oral or nasopharyngeal airway as needed. [See SKILLS] • Maintain cervical spine immobilization if there is evidence of trauma. [See SKILLS] • The airway can swell and close off very quickly in burn patients. Plan for rapid handover/transfer to a provider capable of advanced airway management.

INTRO

ABCDE

TRAUMA

BREATHING

SHOCK

AMS

SKILLS

GLOSSARY

REFS & QUICK CARDS

CONDITION	SIGNS AND SYMPTOMS	IN-DEPTH DESCRIPTION AND MANAGEMENT
Obstruction due to severe allergic reaction (anaphylaxis)	• Mouth, lip, and tongue swelling • Difficulty breathing with stridor and/or wheezing • Rash or hives (patches of pale or red, itchy, warm, swollen skin) • Tachycardia and hypotension • Abnormal sounds from the airway (such as stridor, snoring, gurgling) • Poor chest rise	Severe allergic reactions can cause swelling of the airway that can lead to obstruction. • Give intramuscular adrenaline for airway obstruction, severe wheezing or shock. [See SKILLS] – Adrenaline can wear off in minutes so be prepared to give additional doses. • Place an IV and give IV fluids. [See SKILLS] • Reposition airway as needed (sit patient upright if no trauma) and give oxygen. [See SKILLS] • If severe or not improving, prepare for rapid handover/transfer for advanced airway management.
Obstruction due to trauma	• Neck haematoma or injuries to head and neck • Abnormal sounds from the airway (such as stridor, snoring, gurgling) • Change in voice • Poor chest rise	Airway obstruction may result from injuries to the head or neck. Blood, bone or damaged tissue may block the airway. Penetrating wounds to the neck may also cause obstruction due to swelling or expanding haematoma. • Suction to remove any blood that might block the airway. • Open the airway using jaw thrust only (do not use head-tilt/chin-lift); and place an oral airway as needed (do not use nasopharyngeal airways if there is facial trauma). [See SKILLS} • Maintain cervical spine immobilization if there is evidence of trauma. [See SKILLS] • Plan for rapid handover/transfer to advanced provider capable of advanced airway management or surgical intervention.

For any abnormal airway sounds, re-assess airway frequently as partial obstruction may worsen rapidly and block airway.

BREATHING conditions

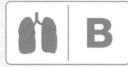

CONDITION	SIGNS AND SYMPTOMS	IN-DEPTH DESCRIPTION AND MANAGEMENT
Tension pneumothorax	Hypotension WITH difficulty in breathing AND any of the following: • distended neck veins • absent breath sounds on affected side • hyperresonance with percussion on affected side [See SKILLS] • tracheal shift away from affected side	Any pneumothorax can become a tension pneumothorax. Air in the cavity between the lungs and the chest wall can collapse the lung (simple pneumothorax). Building pressure (tension) from a large pneumothorax can displace and block flow from the main vessels back to the heart, causing shock (tension pneumothorax). • If tension pneumothorax is suspected, perform emergency needle decompression. [See SKILLS] • Give oxygen. [See SKILLS] • Give IV fluids. [See SKILLS] • Arrange for rapid handover/transfer to an advanced provider capable of placing a chest tube.
Suspected opioid overdose	• Slow respiratory rate • Hypoxia • Very small pupils	Opioid medications (such as morphine, pethidine, and heroin) can decrease the body's drive to breathe. • Give naloxone to reverse the effects of opioids. [See SKILLS] – Monitor closely as naloxone will wear off and additional doses may be needed. • Give oxygen. [See SKILLS]
Asthma/ COPD (chronic obstructive pulmonary disease)	• Wheezing • Cough • Accessory muscle use • May have history of asthma/COPD diagnosis, allergies or smoking	Asthma and COPD are conditions causing spasm in the lower airways, resulting in narrowing that causes difficulty in breathing and wheezing. • Administer salbutamol as soon as possible. (Salbutamol helps to relieve the spasm in the air passages) [See SKILLS] • Give oxygen if indicated. [See SKILLS]
Large pleural effusion/ haemothorax	• Decreased breath sounds on affected side • Dull sounds with percussion on affected side [See SKILLS] • If there is a large amount of fluid, may have shock	Pleural effusion occurs when fluid builds up in the space between the lung and the chest wall or diaphragm. As the fluid builds up, it limits expansion of the lungs. • Give oxygen. [See SKILLS] • Arrange for handover/transfer immediately (many of these patients will need a procedure to drain fluid).

If cause unknown, remember the possibility of trauma [See TRAUMA]

CIRCULATION conditions

CONDITION	SIGNS AND SYMPTOMS	IN-DEPTH DESCRIPTION AND MANAGEMENT
Pulselessness	• No pulse • Unconscious • Not breathing	Follow relevant cardiopulmonary resuscitation (CPR) protocols.
Shock	• Rapid heart rate (tachycardia) • Rapid breathing (tachypnoea) • Pale and cool skin • Capillary refill>3 seconds • Sweating (diaphoresis) • May have dizziness, confusion, altered mental status • May have hypotension	Poor perfusion is the failure to deliver enough oxygen-carrying blood to the vital organs. When poor perfusion continues until organ function is affected, this is called shock and can lead rapidly to death. • Initial treatment for shock includes laying the patient flat (if tolerated). • Give oxygen. [See SKILLS] • Control bleeding. [See SKILLS] • Start an IV and give IV fluids. [See SKILLS] • If there are signs of infection, give antibiotics if available. • Prepare for rapid handover/transfer.

Severe bleeding (haemorrhage)	• Bleeding wounds
	• Bruising around the umbilicus (belly button) or over the flanks can be a sign of internal bleeding
	• Bleeding from the rectum or vagina or in vomit
	• Pelvic fracture
	• Femur fracture
	• Decreased breath sounds on one side of the chest (haemothorax)
	• Signs of poor perfusion (such as hypotension, tachycardia, pale skin, diaphoresis)
		External bleeding that is not controlled can lead quickly to shock. A large quantity of blood can also be lost into the chest, pelvis, thigh and abdomen before the bleeding is recognized.
		• Stop the bleeding. Depending on the source, use:
		  – direct pressure [See SKILLS]
		  – deep wound packing [See SKILLS]
		  – a tourniquet [See SKILLS]
		  – pelvic binder or femur splint. [See SKILLS]
		• Give IV fluids. [See SKILLS]
		• Refer for blood transfusion and ongoing surgical management if needed.
		A tourniquet should be used only for life-threatening bleeding.

Pericardial tamponade	• Signs of poor perfusion (tachycardia, tachypnoea, hypotension, pale and cool skin, cold extremities, capillary refill >3 seconds) • Distended neck veins • Muffled heart sounds • May have dizziness, confusion, altered mental status	Pericardial tamponade occurs when fluid builds up in the sac around the heart. The pressure from this fluid can collapse the chambers of the heart and keep them from filling properly, limiting blood flow to the tissues and causing shock. Treatment is drainage by pericardiocentesis. • In order to keep the patient alive until the fluid around the heart can be drained, give IV fluids to ensure that as much volume as possible enters the heart. [See SKILLS] • Refer rapidly for surgical management.

If cause unknown, remember the possibility of trauma [See TRAUMA]

DISABILITY conditions

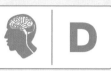

CONDITION	SIGNS AND SYMPTOMS	IN-DEPTH DESCRIPTION AND MANAGEMENT
Hypoglycaemia	• Sweating (diaphoresis) • Altered mental status (ranging from confusion to unconsciousness) • Seizures/convulsions • Blood glucose <3.5 mmol/L • History of diabetes, malaria or severe infection • Responds quickly to glucose	Patients with hypoglycaemia (low blood sugar) need glucose immediately. [See SKILLS] • If the person can speak and swallow, give oral glucose. • If the person cannot speak or is unconscious, give IV glucose if possible. • If IV glucose is not possible or available, give buccal (inside of the cheek) glucose. [See SKILLS]
Increased pressure on the brain	• Headache • Seizures/convulsions • Nausea, vomiting • Altered mental status • Unequal pupils • Weakness on one side of the body	Increased pressure on the brain can occur from trauma, tumours, increased fluid, bleeding or infections. Because the skull is rigid, any swelling, fluid, or mass increases the pressure around the brain, limiting blood flow and possibly displacing brain tissue, causing death. • Raise the head of the bed to 30 degrees if there is no concern for trauma and there is no hypotension. • Check glucose. [See SKILLS] • If there are seizures/convulsions, give a benzodiazepine. [See SKILLS] • The pressure must be reduced as quickly as possible. Arrange for rapid handover/transfer to a surgical centre.
Seizure/ convulsion	Signs and symptoms of active seizure: • Repetitive movements, gaze fixed to one side or alternating rhythmically and not responsive. Sign and symptoms of recent seizure: • Bitten tongue • Urinated on self • Known history of seizures/convulsions • Confusion that gradually improves over minutes to hours	The goal in managing seizures/convulsions is to prevent hypoxia and injury. • Protect the seizing person from falls and from any hard or sharp objects nearby. • Do not place anything in the mouth of a person with active seizure except to suction airway. [See SKILLS] • Give oxygen. [See SKILLS] • Check blood glucose. Give glucose if <3.5 mmol/L. [See SKILLS] • Treat with a benzodiazepine [See SKILLS] and monitor closely for slowing or difficult breathing. • Place patient in recovery position if there is no trauma suspected. [See SKILLS] • If the patient is pregnant, or recently gave birth, give magnesium sulphate. [See SKILLS]

If cause unknown, remember the possibility of trauma [See TRAUMA]

INTRO

ABCDE

TRAUMA

BREATHING

SHOCK

AMS

SKILLS

GLOSSARY

REFS & QUICK CARDS

EXPOSURE conditions

CONDITION	SIGNS AND SYMPTOMS	IN-DEPTH DESCRIPTION AND MANAGEMENT
Snake bite	• History of snake bite • Bite marks may be seen • Oedema • Blistering of the skin • Bruising • Hypotension • Paralysis • Seizures • Bleeding from wounds	The goal of managing snake bites is to limit the spread of the venom and the effects of venom on the body. • Immobilize the extremity. [See SKILLS] • Take a picture of the snake when possible and send with the patient (for example, with the patient's mobile phone). • Give IV fluids if evidence of shock. [See SKILLS] • These patients may have delayed shock or airway problems. Monitor closely and plan early for rapid handover/transfer.

Vital signs should be checked at the end of the ABCDE

A full set of vital signs (blood pressure, heart rate, respiratory rate, and oxygen saturation if available) should be performed after the ABCDE approach. Do not delay ABCDE interventions for vital signs.

ABCDE SHOULD BE REPEATED FREQUENTLY

The ABCDE approach is designed to quickly identify reversible life-threatening conditions. Ideally, the ABCDE approach should be repeated at least every 15 minutes or with any change in condition.

Workbook question 2: ABCDE approach

Using the workbook section above, list the management for airway blocked by a foreign body.

_____

_____

_____

_____

_____

_____

_____

PAEDIATRIC ABCDE CONSIDERATIONS

While the ABCDE approach is used in both adults and children, there are some aspects of assessing and managing children that are different from adults. The "Paediatric considerations" sections throughout the workbook highlight these differences.

Paediatric considerations
Pediatric airway conditions

Excessive drooling, stridor, airway swelling and unwillingness to move the neck are all high-risk signs in children. Look carefully in the airway for foreign bodies, burns or obstruction. Allow the child to remain in a position of comfort. Position airway as needed below.

Compared to adults, children have:	So you must do this:
Bigger tongues.	• Place the child in the "sniffing" position (modified head-tilt, chin-lift – like the slight upward and forward tilt of the head when sniffing a flower).
Shorter necks with airways that are softer and more easily blocked.	• Avoid over-extending or flexing the neck.
A larger head compared to the rest of the body.	• Watch closely for airway obstruction. • Use the jaw thrust if airway is not open. [See SKILLS] • Position head (using padding under shoulders for very small children) to open airway if no trauma. [See SKILLS]

For choking, use age-appropriate chest thrusts/abdominal thrusts/back blows. [See SKILLS]

INTRO
ABCDE
TRAUMA
BREATHING
SHOCK
AMS
SKILLS
GLOSSARY
REFS & QUICK CARDS

Pediatric breathing conditions

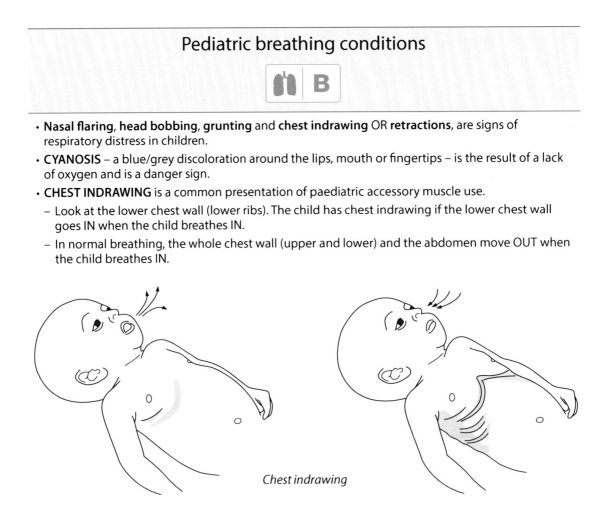

- **Nasal flaring**, **head bobbing**, **grunting** and **chest indrawing** OR **retractions**, are signs of respiratory distress in children.
- **CYANOSIS** – a blue/grey discoloration around the lips, mouth or fingertips – is the result of a lack of oxygen and is a danger sign.
- **CHEST INDRAWING** is a common presentation of paediatric accessory muscle use.
  - Look at the lower chest wall (lower ribs). The child has chest indrawing if the lower chest wall goes IN when the child breathes IN.
  - In normal breathing, the whole chest wall (upper and lower) and the abdomen move OUT when the child breathes IN.

Chest indrawing

- A **SILENT CHEST** (no breath sounds when you listen to the chest) is a sign of severe respiratory distress in a child. With severe spasm and narrowing of the airways, there may be limited air movement and few breath sounds on exam. Give salbutamol and oxygen and re-assess frequently. [See SKILLS]
- **STRIDOR** signals severe airway compromise, and there are many possible causes. Children with stridor should be allowed to stay in a position of comfort and transferred immediately to an advanced provider. Further treatment will often include nebulized adrenaline. If immediate transfer is not possible, consider intramuscular adrenaline as per severe allergic reaction treatment. [See SKILLS]

Pediatric circulation conditions

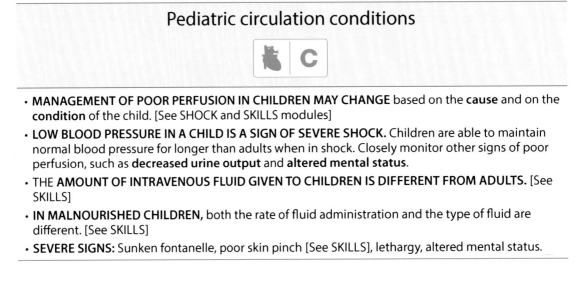

- **MANAGEMENT OF POOR PERFUSION IN CHILDREN MAY CHANGE** based on the **cause** and on the **condition** of the child. [See SHOCK and SKILLS modules]
- **LOW BLOOD PRESSURE IN A CHILD IS A SIGN OF SEVERE SHOCK.** Children are able to maintain normal blood pressure for longer than adults when in shock. Closely monitor other signs of poor perfusion, such as **decreased urine output** and **altered mental status**.
- THE **AMOUNT OF INTRAVENOUS FLUID GIVEN TO CHILDREN IS DIFFERENT FROM ADULTS.** [See SKILLS]
- **IN MALNOURISHED CHILDREN,** both the rate of fluid administration and the type of fluid are different. [See SKILLS]
- **SEVERE SIGNS:** Sunken fontanelle, poor skin pinch [See SKILLS], lethargy, altered mental status.

Pediatric disability conditions

- **LOW BLOOD GLUCOSE** is a very common cause of altered mental status in sick children.
  - If possible, check blood glucose in children with altered mental status.
  - When it is not possible to check the blood glucose level, administer glucose.

- Always check for seizure/convulsions.
- It is sometimes difficult to determine if infants are acting normally. Always ask the person caring for the child.

Pediatric exposure conditions

- **INFANTS AND CHILDREN HAVE DIFFICULTY MAINTAINING TEMPERATURE** and can very quickly become hypothermic (low body temperature) or hyperthermic (high body temperature).
  - Remove wet clothing and dry skin thoroughly. Place infants skin-to-skin when possible.
  - For hypothermia, be sure to cover infants' heads (but do not obstruct face).
  - For hyperthermia, unbundle tightly wrapped infants.

PAEDIATRIC DANGER SIGNS IN ABCDE

In addition to performing a thorough ABCDE approach, all paediatric patients should be evaluated for the presence of danger signs. Children with danger signs need URGENT attention and referral/handover to a provider able to provide advanced paediatric care.

Paediatric danger signs include:

- Signs of airway obstruction (stridor or drooling/unable to swallow saliva)
- Increased breathing effort (fast breathing, nasal flaring, grunting, chest indrawing or retractions)
- Cyanosis (blue colour of the skin, especially at the lips and fingertips)
- Altered mental status (including lethargy or unusual sleepiness, confusion, disorientation)
- Moves only when stimulated or no movement at all (AVPU other than "A")
- Not feeding well or cannot drink or breastfeed
- Vomiting everything
- Seizures/convulsions
- Low body temperature (hypothermia)

INTRO

ABCDE

TRAUMA

BREATHING

SHOCK

AMS

SKILLS

GLOSSARY

REFS & QUICK CARDS

Workbook question 3: ABCDE approach

Using the workbook section above, list one of each of the following:

- **a paediatric airway consideration**

_____

- **a paediatric breathing consideration**

_____

- **a paediatric circulation consideration**

_____

- **a paediatric disability consideration**

_____

- **a paediatric exposure consideration**

_____

Elements of the SAMPLE history

The SAMPLE approach is a standard way of gathering the key history related to an illness or injury. Sources of information include: the ill/injured person, family members, friends, bystanders, or prior providers. SAMPLE stands for:

S: Signs and symptoms

The patient/family's report of signs and symptoms is essential to assessment and management.

A: Allergies

It is important to be aware of medication allergies so that treatments do not cause harm. Allergies may also suggest anaphylaxis as the cause of acute symptoms.

M: Medications

Obtain a full list of medications that the person currently takes and ask about recent medication or dose changes. These may affect treatment decisions and are important to understanding the person's chronic conditions.

P: Past medical history

Knowing prior medical conditions may help in understanding the current illness and may change management choices.

L: Last oral intake

Record the time of last oral intake and whether solid or liquid. A full stomach increases the risk of vomiting and subsequent choking, especially with sedation or intubation that might be required for surgical procedures.

E: Events surrounding the injury or illness

Knowing the circumstances around the injury or illness may be helpful in understanding the cause, progression and severity.

Workbook question 4: SAMPLE history

Using the workbook section above, list what the letters in SAMPLE stand for:

S: _____

A: _____

M: _____

P: _____

L: _____

E: _____

DISPOSITION CONSIDERATIONS

- If you have to intervene in any of the ABCDE categories, immediately plan for handover/transfer to a higher level of care.

- Once you have completed the ABCDE approach, take a SAMPLE history and complete a physical examination based on the specific condition (secondary examination).

- A good handover summary [See SKILLS] to the next provider requires:

  - brief identification of the patient;

  - relevant elements of the SAMPLE history;

  - physical examination findings;

  - record of interventions given;

  - plans for care needed next and other concerns you may have.

INTRO

ABCDE

TRAUMA

BREATHING

SHOCK

AMS

SKILLS

GLOSSARY

REFS & QUICK CARDS

FOR REFERENCE: NORMAL VITAL SIGNS

NORMAL ADULT VITAL SIGNS

- Pulse rate: 60–100 beats per minute
- Respiratory rate: 10–20 breaths per minute
  - A respiratory rate of less than eight breaths per minute is a danger sign and may require intervention.
- Systolic blood pressure >90 mmHg
- Oxygen saturation >92%
- If you cannot take a blood pressure reading, you can use the pulse to estimate systolic blood pressure. Feeling for a pulse at the locations below can provide an estimate of systolic blood pressure in an adult (although this method may not work well in the elderly):
  - Carotid (neck) pulse ≥ 60 mmHg
  - Femoral (groin) pulse ≥ 70 mmHg
  - Radial (wrist) pulse ≥ 80 mmHg

NORMAL PAEDIATRIC VITAL SIGNS

Vital signs are age-dependent in children. Normal heart rate and respiratory rate are higher in younger children, and normal blood pressures are lower. The brachial (middle of the upper arm) artery should be used to check the pulse in infants and small children.

Normal paediatric vital signs

AGE (in years)	NORMAL HEART RATE (beats per minute)
≤1	100–160
1–3	90–150
4–5	80–140

AGE	RESPIRATORY RATE (breaths per minute)
≤2 months	40–60
2–12 months	25–50
1–5 years	20–40

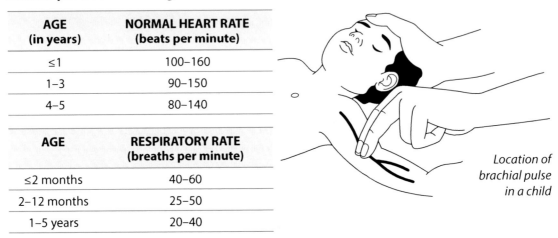

Location of brachial pulse in a child

* To estimate a child's (1–10 years old) weight in kilograms use the formula:

[age in years + 4] x 2

or use weight-estimation tools such as PAWPER, Mercy TAPE, or Broselow tape.

- Children are able to maintain normal blood pressure for longer than adults when they are in shock. You must check closely for signs of poor perfusion.
- The amount of IV fluid appropriate for children is different from that for adults. [See SKILLS]

INTRO

ABCDE

TRAUMA

BREATHING

SHOCK

AMS

SKILLS

GLOSSARY

REFS & QUICK CARDS

FACILITATOR-LED CASE SCENARIOS

These case scenarios will be discussed in small groups. These cases in this module will NOT be assessed and are for practice only. It is important that you practise with these scenarios since you will be assessed on how you lead a case in later modules. To complete a case scenario, the group must identify the critical findings and management needed and formulate a 1–2 line handover summary that includes assessment findings and interventions. You should use the Quick Cards to manage these scenarios.

CASE #1: ADULT ABCDE

A 70-year-old man is brought in by taxi. The driver states the patient lost consciousness while talking with his daughter. There was no trauma, but the daughter poured water on him to try to wake him up. Initially he was confused and vomiting. Now he is unconscious with a respiratory rate of 3 breaths per minute.

1. What do you need to do in your initial approach?

2. Use the ABCDE approach to assess and manage this patient. Ask the facilitator about look, listen and feel findings; use the Quick Card for reference as needed.

	ASSESSMENT	FINDINGS	INTERVENTION NEEDED?		INTERVENTIONS TO PERFORM:
AIRWAY			YES	NO	
BREATHING			YES	NO	
CIRCULATION			YES	NO	
DISABILITY			YES	NO	
EXPOSURE			YES	NO	

3. Formulate 1–2 sentences to summarize this patient for handover.

CASE #2: PAEDIATRIC ABCDE

A mother brings in her 2-year-old son for difficulty in breathing. She reports that he has had a fever for 3 days and has had worsening difficulty in breathing. He has been coughing a lot and today will not eat or drink.

1. What is your initial approach to this patient?

2. Use the ABCDE approach to assess and manage this patient. Ask the facilitator for specific findings when you look, listen and feel; use the Quick Card for reference as needed.

	ASSESSMENT	FINDINGS	INTERVENTION NEEDED?		INTERVENTIONS TO PERFORM:
AIRWAY			YES	NO	
BREATHING			YES	NO	
CIRCULATION			YES	NO	
DISABILITY			YES	NO	
EXPOSURE			YES	NO	

3. Formulate a 1–2 sentence summary of this patient for handover.

MULTIPLE CHOICE QUESTIONS

Answer the questions below. Questions and answers will be discussed within the session.

1. A mother brings in her 3-year-old child because of difficulty in breathing. On assessment, you hear loud, high-pitched sounds when the child breathes in. What is the most immediate concern?

   A. Severe infection

   B. Shock

   C. Asthma attack

   D. Upper airway obstruction

2. An elderly woman fell at home. She had normal vital signs, but complained of neck and knee pain prior to transport. During transport, she starts snoring and gurgling when taking a breath. What is the most appropriate method to immediately manage this problem?

   A. Placing her in the recovery position

   B. Administering salbutamol

   C. Jaw thrust

   D. Head-tilt/chin-lift

PARTICIPANT WORKBOOK

INTRO

ABCDE

TRAUMA

BREATHING

SHOCK

AMS

SKILLS

GLOSSARY

REFS & QUICK CARDS

3. A 50-year-old man has collapsed in a store and you are called to assist him. He is unconscious, has a respiratory rate of four breaths per minute and a pulse of 100 beats per minute. The collapse was witnessed and there is no trauma. What is the best next step?

A. Begin chest compressions

B. Open the airway

C. Begin bag-valve-mask ventilations

D. Check pupils

4. A 2-year-old boy is brought to you for being more sleepy than normal. He is unconscious. You open his airway, and insert an oropharyngeal airway. What is your next step?

A. Check blood pressure

B. Check AVPU scale

C. Check glucose

D. Check breathing

5. You are listening to the lungs of a 26-year-old man who has sudden onset chest pain and he is taking 30 breaths a minute. Which lung-sound finding is most suggestive of pneumothorax?

A. Crackles on both sides

B. Absent lung sounds on one side

C. Stridor

D. Wheezing on both sides

Notes

Module 2: Approach to trauma

Objectives

On completing this module you should be able to:

1. recognize key history findings suggestive of high-risk injuries;

2. recognize physical examination findings suggestive of high-risk injuries;

3. perform Trauma Primary Survey (the ABCDE approach to trauma patients);

4. perform Trauma Secondary Survey (the head-to-toe trauma exam);

5. recognize life-threatening injuries;

6. perform critical interventions for high-risk conditions.

Essential skills

• Cervical spine immobilization	• Direct pressure for haemorrhage control, including deep wound packing
• Spine immobilization and log-roll manoeuvre	• Tourniquet for haemorrhage control
• Jaw-thrust manoeuvre	• IV line insertion
• Airway suctioning	• IV fluid resuscitation
• Insertion of oropharyngeal and nasopharyngeal airway	• AVPU and GCS assessment
• Recovery Position	• Pelvic binding
• Oxygen delivery	• Basic fracture immobilization
• Bag-valve-mask ventilation	• Trauma secondary survey
• Needle decompression for tension pneumothorax	• Basic wound management, including irrigation (washing)
• Three-sided dressing for a sucking chest wound	• Burn management

KEY TERMS

Write the definition using the Glossary at the back of the workbook.

AVPU:

_____

Bradycardia:

_____

Circumferential burn:

_____

Crepitus:

_____

Compartment syndrome:

_____

INTRO

ABCDE

TRAUMA

BREATHING

SHOCK

AMS

SKILLS

GLOSSARY

REFS & QUICK CARDS

Cyanosis:

Decontamination:

Deep wound packing:

Diaphoresis:

Direct pressure:

Disposition:

Escharotomy:

Flail chest:

Fracture:

Glasgow Coma Scale:

Guarding:

Haemorrhage:

Haemorrhagic shock:

Haematoma:

Haemothorax:

Hyperresonance:

Hypothermia:

Hypovolaemic shock:

Hypoxia:

Laceration:

Large bore IV:

Log-roll manoeuvre:

Needle decompression:

Parkland Formula:

Percussion:

Pericardial tamponade:

Pneumothorax:

Priapism:

Rebound tenderness:

SAMPLE history:

Shock:

Sprain:

Sucking chest wound:

Tension pneumothorax:

Trauma primary survey:

Trauma secondary survey:

INTRO

ABCDE

TRAUMA

BREATHING

SHOCK

AMS

SKILLS

GLOSSARY

REFS & QUICK CARDS

Overview

GENERAL PRINCIPLES OF TRAUMA CARE

Early priorities for an injured person include managing airway and breathing emergencies, controlling bleeding, treating shock and immobilizing the spine if needed.

> **The goal of INITIAL ASSESSMENT** is to identify life-threatening injuries.
>
> **The goal of ACUTE MANAGEMENT** is to ensure oxygenation and perfusion, to control pain and to plan ongoing care.

This module will guide you through the:

- Approach to trauma
- ABCDE: Trauma primary survey
- DO: Important conditions to recognize and manage in the primary survey (signs, symptoms and management)
- ASK: Key history findings (SAMPLE history)
- CHECK: Trauma secondary survey
- DO: Important conditions to recognize and manage based on the history and secondary survey (Signs, symptoms and management)
- Special populations
  - Trauma in pregnancy
  - Special considerations in children
- Disposition considerations

APPROACH TO TRAUMA

Approach to the trauma patient consists of three phases:

- **Trauma primary survey:** The ABCDE approach for injured patients
- **SAMPLE history:** Signs and Symptoms, Allergies, Medications, Past medical history, Last oral intake, and Events surrounding the injury
- **Trauma secondary survey:** A complete head-to-toe examination to look for injuries not identified by the primary survey

During primary and secondary surveys, if life-threatening problems are identified, STOP AND MANAGE them.

ABCDE: TRAUMA PRIMARY SURVEY

The ABCDE approach in injured patients is often also called the trauma primary survey. As for all patients this should be conducted within the first 5 minutes and repeated whenever the patient's condition worsens. This trauma-specific ABCDE approach includes the initial assessment and management for all immediately life-threatening injuries. Always suspect head and spine injury in a trauma patient with altered mental status.

	ASSESSMENT	IMMEDIATE MANAGEMENT
Airway with cervical spine immobilization	**Look for:** • blood, vomit, tongue or objects obstructing the airway • burned nasal hairs or soot around the nose or mouth • head or neck trauma • neck haematoma (bleeding under the skin) • altered mental status, as this can affect the ability to protect the airway **Listen for** abnormal airway sounds (such as gurgling, snoring, stridor, noisy breathing).	• Stabilize the cervical spine. [See SKILLS] • Open airway using jaw thrust, NOT head-tilt chin-lift if suspected spine injury. [See SKILLS] • Suction airway secretions, blood and/or vomit. Remove any visible foreign objects from the airway. [See SKILLS] • Place oral airway (avoid nasal airway if facial trauma). [See SKILLS] • If the patient has an expanding neck haematoma or evidence of airway burns or trauma, plan for rapid handover/transfer to a provider capable of advanced airway management. If the airway is open, move onto "Breathing".
Breathing	**Look for:** • increased work of breathing • abnormal chest wall movement which may indicate flail chest • tracheal shift • sucking chest wound • cyanosis (blue-grey color of the skin) around the lips and fingertips • abrasion, bruising or other signs of injury to chest • circumferential burns (burns that go all the way around a body part) to chest or abdomen • absent or decreased breath sounds **Listen for** dull sounds or hyperresonance with percussion. **Feel for** crepitus (cracking and popping when pressing on the skin).	• Give oxygen. [See SKILLS] • Perform needle decompression immediately and give oxygen and IV fluids for tension pneumothorax. [See SKILLS] • Place three-sided dressing for sucking chest wound. [See SKILLS] • If breathing not adequate or patient remains hypoxic on oxygen, assist breathing with bag-valve-mask ventilation. [See SKILLS] • For chest or abdominal burns that restrict breathing, handover for escharotomy (a surgical procedure to cut and release burned tissue that may restrict breathing or blood supply to a limb). If breathing is adequate, move onto "Circulation".

INTRO
ABCDE
TRAUMA
BREATHING
SHOCK
AMS
SKILLS
GLOSSARY
REFS & QUICK CARDS

	ASSESSMENT	IMMEDIATE MANAGEMENT
Circulation	**Look for:** • capillary refill longer than 3 seconds • pale extremities • distended neck veins • external AND internal bleeding Common sources of serious bleeding are: • chest injuries • abdominal injuries • pelvic fractures • femur fractures • amputations or large external wounds • burns, noting size and depth **Feel for:** • cold extremities • weak pulse or tachycardia	• Apply direct pressure to control active bleeding, or deep wound packing if large or gaping. [See SKILLS] • If amputated limbs or any other source of uncontrolled bleeding are present, apply tourniquet (document time of application), start IV fluids and plan for urgent transfer to a surgical unit. [See SKILLS] • If ongoing blood loss or evidence of poor perfusion, place two large bore IVs, give IV fluids and re-assess. [See SKILLS] • If burn injury, start IV fluids according to burn size. • Splint suspected femur fracture. [See SKILLS] • Bind pelvic fracture. [See SKILLS] • Leave any penetrating objects in place and stabilize object for transfer to a surgical team. • Position pregnant patients on their left side while maintaining spinal immobilization. If circulation is adequate, move onto "Disability".
Disability	**Look for:** • confusion, lethargy or agitation • seizures/convulsions • unequal or poorly reactive pupils • deformities of skull • blood or fluid from ear or nose **Check:** • AVPU or GCS • movement and sensation in all extremities • blood glucose level if confused or unconscious	• If GCS <9 (or for children, AVPU score of P or U), plan for rapid handover/transfer to a provider capable of advanced airway management. • If patient is lethargic or unconscious, re-assess the airway frequently as above. • Suspect spine injury or closed head injury with any trauma and altered mental status. • Give oxygen if concern for hypoxia as a cause of altered mental status. [See SKILLS] • Give glucose if altered mental status and: measured low blood glucose, unable to check blood glucose, or history of diabetes. [See SKILLS] • If seizing, give a benzodiazepine. [See SKILLS]

	ASSESSMENT	IMMEDIATE MANAGEMENT
Exposure 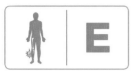	Remove all clothing. Examine entire body for evidence of injury (including the back, spine, groin and underarms) using the log-roll manoeuvre.	• If spinal injury is suspected, perform log-roll manoeuvre to examine the back. [See SKILLS] • Remove restrictive clothing and all jewellery. • Remove any wet clothes and dry patient thoroughly. • Cover the patient as soon as possible to prevent hypothermia. Acutely injured patients have difficulty regulating body temperature. • Respect the patient and protect modesty during exposure.

Workbook question 1: Approach to trauma

A middle-aged man is brought in after being hit by a car. Using the workbook section above, list the immediate management for the assessment findings below.

PRIMARY SURVEY FINDINGS	IMMEDIATE MANAGEMENT
On airway assessment: • Gurgling airway sounds • Obvious head trauma	1. _____ 2. _____ 3. _____ 4. _____
On circulation assessment: • Weak pulses • Capillary refill of <3 seconds • Unstable pelvis on exam	1. _____ 2. _____ 3. _____

INTRO

ABCDE

TRAUMA

BREATHING

SHOCK

AMS

SKILLS

GLOSSARY

REFS & QUICK CARDS

DO: IMPORTANT CONDITIONS TO RECOGNIZE AND MANAGE IN THE PRIMARY SURVEY

	A	Airway conditions

CONDITION	SIGNS AND SYMPTOMS	IN-DEPTH MANAGEMENT

Airway obstruction	• Visible blood, secretions, vomit, tongue or foreign bodies in the airway
	• Changes in voice
	• Abnormal sounds from the airway (such as stridor, snoring, gurgling)
	• Neck haematoma or burns to head and neck
	• Mental status changes leading to airway obstruction
	• Poor chest rise
	• Injury causing swelling of the airway (such as anaphylaxis or airway burn)
		Head and neck injuries may result in obstruction of the airway by blood, secretions, vomit, foreign bodies, or swelling. Penetrating wounds to the neck can cause expanding haematomas. Inhalational injuries due to burns can cause swelling.
		
		• Patients with a decreased level of consciousness may not be able to protect their airways and need to be watched for vomiting and aspiration.
		  – Suction the airway and remove foreign bodies.
		  – Open the airway using a jaw thrust manoeuvre (NOT head-tilt/chin-lift) and place an oral airway as needed. [See: SKILLS]
		• Maintain cervical spine immobilization throughout, if needed.
		• Plan for rapid handover/transfer to a provider capable of advanced airway management.

	B	Breathing conditions

CONDITION	SIGNS AND SYMPTOMS	IN-DEPTH MANAGEMENT

Tension pneumothorax	• Hypotension WITH:
	  – difficulty breathing
	  – distended neck veins
	  – absent breath sounds on affected side
	  – hyperresonance with percussion on affected side
	  – may have tracheal shift away from affected side
		Any pneumothorax can become a tension pneumothorax. Air in the cavity between the lungs and the chest wall can collapse the lung (simple pneumothorax). Building pressure (tension) from a large pneumothorax can displace and block flow from the great vessels to the heart, causing shock as the heart cannot receive and pump enough blood to the rest of the body (tension pneumothorax). In tension pneumothorax, perfusion is compromised.
		
		• Treat tension pneumothorax immediately with needle depression. [See: SKILLS]
		• Give oxygen and IV fluids. [See: SKILLS]
		• Plan for rapid handover/transfer to an advanced provider capable of placing a chest tube.

CONDITION	SIGNS AND SYMPTOMS	IN-DEPTH MANAGEMENT

Sucking chest wound (open pneumothorax)	• Open wound in the chest wall with air passing through causing bubbling or "sucking" noises
	• Difficulty in breathing
	• Chest pain
		Sucking chest wounds are important to recognize because they can rapidly cause a tension pneumothorax. Air enters the chest cavity (into the space between the chest wall and the lungs) through the wound in the chest wall when the patient takes a breath. Pressure on the lung builds if the air cannot escape.
		• Give oxygen. [See SKILLS]
		• Place a three-sided dressing that allows air to leave with exhalation but prevents air from entering when the person inhales. [See SKILLS]
		  – There is a danger of the dressing becoming stuck to the chest wall with clotted blood and causing a tension pneumothorax.
		  – After applying a three-sided dressing the patient should be observed continuously.
		  – Remove the dressing if worsening respiratory status or evidence of worsening perfusion.
		Plan for rapid handover/transfer to an advanced provider capable of placing a chest tube.

Flail chest	• Difficulty in breathing • Chest pain • Part of chest wall moving in the opposite direction of the rest of the chest when breathing	Flail chest segments occur when ribs are broken in multiple places, freeing an entire section of ribs from the chest wall. Without the connection to the chest wall, this section will move abnormally with breathing and prevent part of the lung from expanding. Flail chest is also usually associated with damage to underlying lung tissue. • Give oxygen and pain control. [See SKILLS] • There is a very high risk of developing difficulty in breathing and hypoxia. • Plan for rapid handover/transfer to a provider capable of chest tube placement, advanced airway placement and ventilation.
Haemothorax	• Difficulty in breathing • Decreased breath sounds on affected side • Dull sounds with percussion on affected side • Large haemothorax may cause shock	Haemothorax (blood in the space between the lungs and the chest wall) can present with decreased or absent breath sounds and dull sounds with percussion on the affected side. • Give oxygen and IV fluids. • Plan for rapid handover/transfer to a centre with surgical capacity.

INTRO

ABCDE

TRAUMA

BREATHING

SHOCK

AMS

SKILLS

GLOSSARY

REFS & QUICK CARDS

C   Circulation conditions

CONDITION	SIGNS AND SYMPTOMS	IN-DEPTH MANAGEMENT
Hypovolaemic shock	• Tachycardia, tachypnoea, pale skin, cold extremities, slow capillary refill • May have dizziness, confusion or altered mental status • May have hypotension • External bleeding or internal bleeding (chest, abdomen, pelvis, femur, blood vessels)	Hypovolaemic shock can result from rapid loss of blood (haemorrhagic shock) or from the fluid loss associated with burns. An adult patient in shock may have only tachycardia (elevated heart rate) and/or tachypnoea (high respiratory rate) and may not have low blood pressure until the condition is immediately life-threatening. Even with a systolic blood pressure greater than 90 mmHg, suspect hypovolaemic shock if there is severe bleeding or any sign of poor perfusion (such as cool, moist, or pale skin, slow capillary refill, fast breathing, confusion, restlessness, anxiety). • Stop bleeding with direct pressure, deep wound packing if wound is gaping, a tourniquet, splinting of fractures and binding the pelvis as needed. [See SKILLS] • Start two large-bore IV lines and give IV fluids. [See SKILLS] • Patients with suspected large haemothorax or other internal haemorrhage will need rapid handover/transfer to a unit with surgical care and blood transfusion capabilities.

REMEMBER... Children and young people are able to maintain a normal blood pressure until they have lost up to a quarter of their blood. Always check for other signs of shock.

[See "Special considerations in children" section]

Pericardial tamponade	• Signs of poor perfusion (such as tachycardia, tachypnoea, hypotension, pale skin, cold extremities, capillary refill greater than 3 seconds) • Distended neck veins • Muffled heart sounds • May have dizziness, confusion, altered mental status	Pericardial tamponade occurs when fluid builds up in the sac around the heart. The pressure from this fluid can collapse the chambers of the heart and prevent them from filling, limiting the amount of blood the heart can pump. • Give IV fluid to improve heart filling. [See SKILLS] • Patients need immediate handover/transfer to an advanced provider for drainage of the fluid.

INTRO

ABCDE

TRAUMA

BREATHING

SHOCK

AMS

SKILLS

GLOSSARY

REFS & QUICK CARDS

D Disability conditions

CONDITION	SIGNS AND SYMPTOMS	IN-DEPTH MANAGEMENT
Severe head injury	• Visual changes, loss of memory, seizures/convulsions, vomiting, headache • Altered mental status or other neurologic deficit • Scalp wound and/or skull deformity • Bruising to head (particularly around eyes or behind ears) • Blood or fluid from the ears or nose • Unequal pupils • Weakness on one side of the body	Brain injuries can range from mild bruising to severe bleeding in or around the brain. Because the skull is rigid, the bleeding cannot expand and causes increased pressure on the brain. If the pressure becomes too high, it will prevent blood from entering into the skull and perfusing the brain, and can squeeze part of the brain through the base of the skull, causing death. Any trauma to the brain can cause significant impact on function. • Always remember that head injuries can be associated with spinal injuries. Immobilize the spine and use the log-roll technique to examine the back of the body. • Use the Glasgow Coma Scale (or AVPU in children) to assess and monitor patients with head injury. • Be sure to frequently re-assess ABCDE. • If concern for open skull fracture, give IV antibiotics as per local protocol. • Always check glucose and administer as needed. • Do not give food or drink by mouth. • Plan for early handover/transfer to a facility with specialist care.

REMEMBER... People who initially appear well may have hidden life-threatening injuries, such as internal bleeding. It is very important to re-assess trauma patients frequently using the primary survey. Once you find a primary survey problem and manage it, go back and repeat the primary survey to identify any new problems and make sure that the management worked. Ideally, the ABCDE approach should be rechecked every 15 minutes and with any change in condition.

Vital signs should be checked at the end of the primary survey

A full set of vital signs (blood pressure, heart rate, respiratory rate and oxygen saturation if available) should be performed after the primary survey. Do not delay primary survey interventions for vital signs.

Workbook question 2: Approach to trauma

Using the workbook section above, list five important conditions to recognize in the primary survey

1. _____

2. _____

3. _____

4. _____

5. _____

ASK: KEY HISTORY FINDINGS FOR TRAUMA PATIENTS

Information about an injured person and the injury event can be critical to planning management. Children, older adults and people with chronic disease have an increased risk of complications from trauma. They may need to be watched for several hours even when they appear well. Certain mechanisms are often associated with multiple injuries, some of which may not be obvious right away. High-risk mechanisms include:

- pedestrian being hit by a vehicle;

- motorcycle crashes or any vehicle crash with unrestrained occupants;

- falls from heights greater than 3 metres (or in children, twice the child's height);

- gunshot or stab wounds;

- and explosion or fire in an enclosed space.

Use the SAMPLE approach to obtain a history. Remember that you may be able to obtain information from bystanders, family, police, fire service or other health-care workers.

If the history identifies a primary survey condition, STOP AND RETURN IMMEDIATELY TO PRIMARY SURVEY to manage it.

S: SIGNS AND SYMPTOMS

- **Is there a history of hoarse or raspy voice, or other voice changes?**
  Changes in voice in the setting of injury to the head, neck or with burns may suggest that the airway is swelling and that it may obstruct.

- **Is there any difficulty in breathing?**
  Problems with breathing may develop over time and might not be present in the initial primary survey. Difficulty in breathing may suggest that the person has an injury to the lungs, ribs, muscles, chest wall or spine.

- **Is there reported bleeding?**

  It is usually quite difficult for patients to estimate the volume of blood loss, but it may be helpful to know how long there has been bleeding, how many bandages have been soaked and if the bleeding is getting lighter or heavier.

- **Is there confusion or unusual sleepiness?**

  Confusion after injury may be a sign of head injury, lack of oxygen or shock (with decreased blood flow to the brain). A head injury can cause bleeding or increased pressure on the brain leading to confusion, lethargy (increased sleepiness) and coma.

- **Is there pain? Where is the pain, what does it feel like and how severe is it?**

  Pain is a sign of underlying injury. Headache may suggest that the person has an injury to the skull or the brain. Pain along the spine can suggest an injury that may progress to cause damage to the spinal cord. Pain in the chest or abdomen may suggest damage to the heart, lungs or other organs. Pain in the pelvis or hips may suggest a fracture in the pelvis which can cause serious bleeding and shock. Pain may be the first sign of an internal injury in the chest, abdomen or pelvis.

- **Is there nausea or vomiting?**

  This may indicate an abdominal or head injury.

- **Is there reported numbness or weakness?**

  This may indicate a spinal injury.

- **Are there reported vision changes?**

  Direct trauma to the eye, fractures of bones around the eye, and head injuries can all cause vision changes.

A: ALLERGIES

- **Any allergies to medications?**

M: MEDICATIONS

- **Currently taking any medications?**

  Medications that affect blood clotting (e.g. aspirin, warfarin, clopidigrel) can make bleeding more difficult to control and increase the risk of delayed bleeding. Blood pressure medications can make it hard to manage shock. Obtain a full list of medications if possible or ask family members to bring in medications.

INTRO

ABCDE

TRAUMA

BREATHING

SHOCK

AMS

SKILLS

GLOSSARY

REFS & QUICK CARDS

P: PAST MEDICAL HISTORY

- **Is the person pregnant?**

  Pregnancy causes some of the organs to be moved out of their usual position and causes changes in the body that need to be considered when managing trauma. Always ask women of childbearing age about the date of last menstrual period.

- **Tetanus status?**

  A person who has not had a tetanus vaccination within the past 5 years and who has an injury that damages the skin needs a tetanus vaccination.

- **Are other conditions present that put the person at higher risk for serious injury?**

  RISK FACTORS FOR POOR OUTCOMES FROM INJURY:

  - Age less than 5 years or greater than 55 years
  - Heart or lung disease
  - Diabetes
  - Liver failure (cirrhosis)
  - Severely overweight
  - Pregnancy
  - Immunosuppression (including HIV)
  - Bleeding disorder or taking blood-thinning medications (medications that prevent clotting)

L: LAST ORAL INTAKE

- **When did the person last eat or drink?**

E: EVENTS SURROUNDING INJURY

Certain mechanisms of injury are so high risk that patients should be observed closely, even if they do not appear to be significantly injured.

- **Was there a fall from 3 metres or more (or twice the height in children)?**

  Falls are a common cause of injury for both adults and children. A greater distance fallen increases the chance of serious injury. Falls in adults are often associated with older age, alcohol intoxication, or the failure of workplace equipment, including scaffolding and ladders. Children often fall from trees, windows or balconies.

- **Was a pedestrian or a cyclist hit by a vehicle?**

  Adults and children who are hit by a vehicle while walking or using non-motorized forms of transport (such as bicycles) are always at high risk of serious injury. Young children may be less able than adults to report events, even major events like being hit by a vehicle. Always consider the possibility of unwitnessed trauma in young children. Children and adults can sustain multiple injuries when hit by a vehicle – both from direct impact to the body, especially the lower extremities, and from secondary impact if they are thrown against the windscreen or road, which may cause injuries anywhere in the body, including to head, neck, chest or limbs.

INTRO

ABCDE

TRAUMA

BREATHING

SHOCK

AMS

SKILLS

GLOSSARY

REFS & QUICK CARDS

- **In a motorcycle (or powered 3-wheeler) crash, was the rider thrown?**

  Motorcycles collisions often result in a rider being thrown. Ask if the motorcyclist was wearing a helmet and how far away from the vehicle the rider was found. Common injury sites include head (especially when no helmet was worn), spine, chest, abdomen and pelvis (as the rider hits the handlebars), as well as limbs and skin (as the rider hits the road).

- **Was there a road traffic crash at high speed? Was the person thrown from or trapped inside a vehicle? Did any vehicle occupants die in this crash?**

  With higher-speed crashes, greater force is transmitted to vehicle occupants increasing the risk of serious injury. Vehicle occupants may be injured by impact with the windscreen or steering wheel, or by the forces that result from the sudden stopping of the vehicle. A person thrown from a vehicle is at very high risk of serious injury. If a person was trapped within a vehicle it is important to find out what part of the body was trapped (arm/leg, etc.) and for how long. Consider crush injury in a person who has been trapped. A death at the scene of a road traffic crash suggests that there was significant force exerted on the vehicle and its passengers. All passengers involved in the crash, even if they appear unhurt, are at high risk for serious injury.

- **In a motor vehicle crash, was the patient wearing a seatbelt?**

  Some types of injuries are more common in patients who were not wearing a seat-belt (being thrown from the vehicle, head strike on the windscreen, chest strike on the steering column). However, in very high-speed crashes, seat belts can also cause certain types of injuries (cervical spine injury, abdominal injury).

- **Was a weapon used?**

  Any time there is a history of a stab or gunshot wound, there may be multiple wounds. Always check the full body for wounds. After a bullet enters the body it may not follow a direct path and can twist throughout the body. Many internal organs can be injured by a single bullet. A stab wound creates a direct path (it is important to know the length of the blade that was used). Remember that blunt injuries from objects such as sticks and bats can cause damage to internal organs in addition to obvious injuries such as fractures, bruises and lacerations.

- **Was there a burn? If so, what type of burn was it?**

  Burns from fires (flame burns) are the most common. A history of flame burn in an enclosed space can also suggest an inhalation or airway injury. Scald burns (due to hot liquids) are common in children. Electrical injuries often come from high-voltage sources such as overhead electrical wires coming in contact with the body. On the surface, these electrical injuries may look small but they can cause extensive tissue and muscle damage. The electrical current often crosses the body, taking the shortest path from the point of contact with the skin to the ground, often leaving entry and exit burn marks. In the case of chemical burns, information about the specific chemical may be needed to remove it properly.

- **For burns, was first aid provided at the scene?**

  It is important to know if the burning process was stopped, and in the event of a chemical exposure, if decontamination was performed. If the burn is less than 3 hours old and no first aid was provided, the wound will need to be washed with clean water to stop the burning process. If there is a history of chemical exposure, protect yourself from the chemical and ensure that it is properly removed from the skin.

- **Did the person sustain a crush injury? Is there severe pain or numbness? Is there dark urine?**

  Crush injuries may damage skin, muscle, blood vessels and bone. Damaged muscle can release a muscle by-product (called myoglobin) that can build up and damage the kidneys. It is important to know how long a body part was crushed. Even a small crushed area can cause the release of a dangerous amount of myoglobin (for example when a limb is caught under falling debris for an extended time). If a person with a crush injury has dark urine, this may be a sign of build-up of myoglobin in the kidneys. Tissue damage and swelling from crush injury can also cause a build-up of pressure (particularly in limb-crush injuries) that can limit blood flow to the muscles and nerves (compartment syndrome).

- **Did the person sustain a blast injury?**

  Blast injuries (from explosions) can involve all systems of the body, especially the hollow organs. Common blast injuries include damage to the lungs, intestines and ears. Patients involved in explosions need to be checked carefully and repeatedly because these injuries are easily missed. Blasts may also be associated with foreign bodies in the skin and eyes, burns or chemical injury, and toxin or radiation exposure.

Workbook question 3: Approach to trauma

Using the workbook section above, list five questions you would ask when taking a SAMPLE history from a person injured in a road traffic crash:

1. _____

2. _____

3. _____

4. _____

5. _____

CHECK: TRAUMA SECONDARY SURVEY

Following the primary survey and SAMPLE history, the secondary survey is a detailed head-to-toe **examination** designed to identify any additional injuries or issues requiring intervention. The secondary survey gives the provider an organized way to assess the entire body for signs of trauma that may not have been obvious on the primary survey. Remember that very painful or frightening injuries may distract both patients and providers from recognising other injuries. Always examine the entire body. If the secondary survey identifies a primary survey condition, **STOP AND RETURN IMMEDIATELY TO THE PRIMARY SURVEY to manage it.**

INTRO

ABCDE

TRAUMA

BREATHING

SHOCK

AMS

SKILLS

GLOSSARY

REFS & QUICK CARDS

Head, ears, eyes, nose, and throat (HEENT)	**Look for:**
	• Scalp wounds or bruising
	• Skull deformities
	• Blood in mouth or throat
	• Unequal or unresponsive pupils indicating head injury
	• Vision loss or changes and eye injuries
	• Any problems with eye movements
	• Blood or fluid from ear or nose, which can indicate tissue injury or skull fracture
	• Tooth injury or poor alignment of teeth
	• Signs of airway burns: ash, singed nasal hairs, new or worsening lip/mouth swelling
	Listen for:
	• Stridor which could indicate that the airway will obstruct soon
	• Gurgling indicating fluid in the airway
	• Changes in voice, which can indicate airway or vocal cord injury
	Feel for:
	• Tenderness or abnormal movement of facial bones, suggesting fracture
	• Loose teeth that may accidentally be inhaled
	• Defects or crepitus in the skull or facial bones concerning for fracture
Neck	**Look for:**
	• Reduced ability to move neck or pain on movement
	• Bruising, bleeding or swelling
	• Haematoma (bruising/bleeding under the skin) – this may eventually cause airway obstruction
	• Penetrating neck wounds
	• Distended neck veins (which may indicate tension pneumothorax or tamponade)
	Feel for:
	• Air in the skin or soft tissue – concerning for airway injury or pneumothorax
	• Tenderness or deformity along the spine – concerning for fracture
Chest	**Look for:**
	• Bruising, deformity, wounds
	• Uneven chest wall movement–concerning for pneumothorax or flail chest
	• Burns around the entire chest (circumferential) which can cause difficulty in breathing
	Listen for:
	• Breath sounds (decreased, unequal or absent, wheeze, crepitations)
	• Muffled heart sounds – concerning for pericardial tamponade
	Feel for:
	• Tenderness
	• Crepitus – concerning for fracture or pneumothorax

Abdomen	**Look for:**
	• Abdominal distension
	• Visible abdominal wounds, bruising or abrasions
	• Bruising on back or abdomen, which may indicate internal bleeding
	• Circumferential burns to the abdomen (may cause severe problems with breathing)
	Feel for:
	• Abdominal rebound tenderness (pain when releasing pressure on the abdomen) or guarding (sudden contraction of the abdominal wall muscles when the abdomen is pressed), suggesting serious injury
	• Abdominal tenderness, which can indicate organ or blood vessel injury
Pelvis and genitals (always protect patient privacy during exam)	**Look for:**
	• Bruising/lacerations to pelvis
	• Blood at the opening of the penis or rectum. May be a sign of sexual assault.
	• Vaginal lacerations or bleeding – these could indicate open pelvic fracture, injury to the uterus, or may be a source of significant blood loss. May be a sign of sexual assault.
	• Penile lacerations
	• Priapism (prolonged erection) can indicate spinal injury
	• Urine colour changes (dark urine or obvious blood) that might indicate muscle breakdown or kidney injury
	Feel for:
	• Tenderness or abnormal movement in pelvis
Extremities	**Look for:**
	• Swelling or bruising
	• Deformity, which could indicate fracture
	• Open fractures
	• Amputation
	• Circumferential burns
	• Pale skin that could indicate limited blood flow
	Feel for:
	• Absent or weak pulses
	• Cold skin that could indicate limited blood flow
	• Tenderness
	• Abnormally firm, painful muscular compartments in the extremities can indicate compartment syndrome

Spine/back	*Log roll the person with assistance, then:*
	Look for:
	• Bruising
	• Deformity
	Feel for:
	• Tenderness, crepitus and alignment along the entire spine (upper neck to lower back)
	• Tenderness, crepitus or misalignment over any other areas with visible evidence of trauma
Skin	**Look for:**
	• Bruising
	• Abrasions
	• Lacerations
	• Feel for peripheral pulses in all extremities
	• Burns
	– Look for circumferential burns: depending on the location, these can cause difficulty in breathing (if on the chest) or compartment syndrome (if on the extremities)
Neurologic	**Check for:**
	• Decreased level of consciousness (using AVPU or GCS) and seizures/convulsions, which may be signs of serious head injury
	• Movement and strength in each limb
	• Sensation on face, chest, abdomen, limbs; if there is a sensory deficit, identify where it begins
	• Priapism (persistent penile erection)
	• Decreased sensation, decreased strength or priapism can indicate spinal cord injury

INTRO
ABCDE
TRAUMA
BREATHING
SHOCK
AMS
SKILLS
GLOSSARY
REFS & QUICK CARDS

Workbook question 4: Approach to trauma

Using the workbook section above, list one way that you would ASSESS the following systems.

Head, ears, eyes, nose, throat:

Listen for: _____

Look for: _____

Feel for: _____

Chest:

Look for: _____

Listen for: _____

Feel for: _____

Pelvis and genitals:

Look for: _____

Feel for: _____

DO: IMPORTANT CONDITIONS TO RECOGNIZE AND MANAGE BASED ON HISTORY AND SECONDARY SURVEY

Management of specific injuries found during secondary survey

CONDITION	SIGNS AND SYMPTOMS	IN-DEPTH MANAGEMENT
Head injury	• Headache • Altered mental status • Abnormal pupils • Scalp lacerations and/or skull fractures • Bruising to head (particularly around eyes or behind ears) • Blood or clear fluid coming from nose or ears • Weakness on one side of the body • Seizures/convulsions • Visual change • Loss of memory • Vomiting	Because the brain is encased in the rigid skull, any swelling or bleeding caused by brain injury can rapidly become life-threatening. • Monitor level of consciousness (a marker of brain function) using the Glasgow Coma Scale (GCS) or AVPU scale in children. [See SKILLS] • Any patient who has significant head injuries is at risk of having spine injuries as well. [See SKILLS] • Always monitor immobilized patients for vomiting to avoid choking. • If there is concern for an open skull fracture, give IV antibiotics. • Check blood glucose and give glucose if less than 3.5 mmol/L or unable to measure. • Any patient with GCS less than 9 should be transferred for a CT scan within 2 hours of injury, if possible.
Facial fractures	• Deformities or unusual movement in the facial bones • Patient reports jaw not closing normally or teeth not aligned • Problems with eye movements	• Give antibiotics for open facial fractures (laceration over a broken bone). • Update tetanus vaccination. • Suspect cervical spine injury and immobilize the cervical spine if needed. [See SKILLS] • Remember to position patient to keep blood from flowing into airway. • Avoid nasopharyngeal airways and nasogastric tubes when facial fracture is suspected.
Penetrating eye injury	• Any visible object in the eye • Painful red eye or a reported feeling of something in the eye; it may be difficult to see small objects that have penetrated the eye • Problems with vision • An abnormally shaped pupil or clear liquid draining from the eye may indicate a puncture wound • Evidence of facial trauma	• Avoid any pressure on the injured eye – this could worsen the injury • Do not remove objects penetrating the eye. • Give antibiotics. • Update tetanus vaccination if needed. • Keep the head elevated and place a loose patch over both eyes (do NOT put pressure on the eye). • Plan for handover/transfer to an advanced provider.

INTRO
ABCDE
TRAUMA
BREATHING
SHOCK
AMS
SKILLS
GLOSSARY
REFS & QUICK CARDS

Management of specific injuries found during secondary survey

CONDITION	SIGNS AND SYMPTOMS	IN-DEPTH MANAGEMENT
Penetrating neck wound	• Small lacerations or puncture wounds may be the only sign of serious injury • Swelling (suggesting haematoma) • Look carefully for penetrating objects	Patients with penetrating neck wounds are at risk of airway obstruction, so monitor the airway closely. Neck wounds may also have significant haemorrhage. • Maintain cervical spine precautions. [See SKILLS] • Stabilize, but do not remove penetrating objects. • Apply firm pressure to bleeding site, being careful not to block the airway. • Do not insert anything into wound to check the depth – this can cause further damage. • Initiate rapid handover/transfer to a unit with surgical care and advanced airway management capabilities.
Chest injury	• Difficulty in breathing • Crepitus or tenderness to palpation over the ribs • Uneven chest wall movement or unequal breath sounds	Monitor closely for difficulty in breathing due to lung injury which can develop over time. Tension pneumothorax is treated in the primary survey; however, chest injury may also be associated with simple pneumothorax which can progress to a tension pneumothorax. • Any patient with a pneumothorax should be placed on oxygen and monitored closely for development of a tension pneumothorax. • Crepitus or tenderness may be signs of rib fractures which are often associated with underlying chest or abdominal injury. • Plan for handover/transfer for chest tube (pneumothorax) or advanced airway and breathing management.

Abdominal injury	• Abdominal pain or vomiting
	• Tender, firm or distended abdomen on examination
	• Sudden abdominal wall muscle contractions when the abdomen is touched (guarding)
	• Very few or no bowel sounds on examination
	• Rectal bleeding
	• Visible wound in the abdominal wall
	• Bruising around the umbilicus or over the flanks can be a sign of internal bleeding
		Severe pain or bruising to the abdomen is concerning for organ injury or internal bleeding.
		
		• If you suspect abdominal injuries, give IV fluids.
		• Do not give the patient anything to eat or drink.
		• If bowel is visible:
		  – leave it outside the body;
		  – cover it with sterile gauze soaked in sterile saline;
		  – give antibiotics.
		• If there is any concern for abdominal injury, plan for rapid handover/transfer to a unit with surgical capabilities.

INTRO

ABCDE

TRAUMA

BREATHING

SHOCK

AMS

SKILLS

GLOSSARY

REFS & QUICK CARDS

Management of specific injuries found during secondary survey

CONDITION	SIGNS AND SYMPTOMS	IN-DEPTH MANAGEMENT

Spinal cord injury	• Midline spinal pain/tenderness
	• Movement problems: paralysis, weakness, abnormal reflexes
	• Sensation problems: tingling ("pins and needles" sensation), loss of sensation
	• Loss of control of urine or stool
	• Priapism
	• May have hypotension, bradycardia
	• Crepitus when you touch the spinal bones
	• Spinal bones that are not properly aligned
	• Difficulty in breathing (upper cervical spine injury)
		• Provide spinal immobilization to any person with a history of trauma who is unconscious; or who is conscious and has neck pain, cervical spine tenderness, numbness or weakness.
		  – Use a rolled sheet or neck collar to immobilize the cervical spine. [See SKILLS]
		    ▪ Keep the patient lying flat in bed to immobilize the rest of the spine. [See SKILLS]
		    ▪ When examining or moving the trauma patient, the spine should be protected by using the log-roll manoeuvre. [See SKILLS]
		• Give IV fluids. [See SKILLS]
		• Any patient with possible spinal trauma needs handover/transfer to a specialist unit.

NOTES:

• Spinal trauma is not always obvious. Fractured spinal bones can injure the spinal cord, causing paralysis. If the spinal cord injury is in the cervical spine, paralysis could involve the muscles that control respiration and could lead to death. *Examination findings should be carefully documented so that future providers can evaluate if the patient's condition has changed.*

• Spinal injuries can also cause shock. This can occur when nerves that control the contraction of the blood vessels in the body are damaged. When the walls of a blood vessel relax, the vessel dilates and pressure drops, leading to poor perfusion and shock. Risk is higher if there is also blood loss, so patients must be monitored closely. Always consider spinal injury in a patient with shock that does not improve with treatment.

• Spine boards should only be used to move patients. Leaving patients on spine boards for long periods of time can cause pressure sores. Remove patients from boards as soon as they arrive at the facility and can be laid flat.

CONDITION	SIGNS AND SYMPTOMS	IN-DEPTH MANAGEMENT
Internal bleeding (not seen on primary survey)	• Bruising around the umbilicus or over the flanks can be a sign of internal bleeding • Pelvic fracture • Femur fracture • Decreased breath sounds on one side in the chest (haemothorax) • Signs of poor perfusion (hypotension, tachycardia, pale skin, diaphoresis)	A large quantity of blood can be lost into the chest, pelvis, thigh, and into the abdomen before bleeding is recognized. • Stop the bleeding if possible – bind pelvis or splint femur. [See SKILLS] • Give IV fluid. [See SKILLS] • Refer for blood transfusion and ongoing surgical management if needed.

Management of specific injuries found during secondary survey

CONDITION	SIGNS AND SYMPTOMS	IN-DEPTH MANAGEMENT
Pelvic fracture	• Pain with palpation of the pelvis • Instability or abnormal movement of the pelvic bones • Blood at opening of the penis or rectum	• Give IV fluids and pain control. [See SKILLS] • Compress pelvis gently to check for stability. • Do not open and rock pelvis or perform repeat exams as this can worsen internal bleeding. • Stabilize the pelvis with a sheet or pelvic binder. [See SKILLS] • Plan for early handover/transfer to a unit with blood transfusion capabilities.

Extremity fracture with poor perfusion	• Deformity or crepitus of the bone
	• Absent pulses beyond the fracture
	• Capillary refill time of greater than 3 seconds beyond the fracture
	• Cold extremities beyond the fracture with blue or grey skin colour
		Fractures can displace blood vessels and limit blood supply to the limb beyond the fracture.
		• Look for signs of poor perfusion beyond the fracture.
		  ▪ Feel the pulse.
		  ▪ Check capillary refill.
		  ▪ Look for pale skin. [See SKILLS]
		  ▪ If a fracture is found with weak pulses or poor perfusion, re-establish perfusion by reducing (manually re-aligning bone ends to put limb back to its normal position) and splinting the fracture. [See SKILLS]
		  ▪ Always check and document pulses, capillary refill and sensation before and after any reduction.
		• Plan for urgent handover/transfer to a specialist unit.

Open fracture	• Deformity or crepitus of the bone with overlying laceration	Consider any patient to have an open fracture if there is a wound (more than just a skin abrasion) near a fracture site. Open fractures are emergencies because they can lead to severe bone infections. • Control haemorrhage with direct pressure. [See SKILLS] • Reduce the fracture immediately if there is poor perfusion. [See SKILLS] • Irrigate the wound well. [See SKILLS] • Dress wound. • Give antibiotics and tetanus vaccination. • Splint the wound. • Plan for handover/transfer to a specialist unit.

Management of specific injuries found during secondary survey

CONDITION	SIGNS AND SYMPTOMS	IN-DEPTH MANAGEMENT
Open wound	• Laceration • Abrasion • Wounds in the underarm area, genital area, buttocks or back are easily missed • Pumping or squirting blood can indicate arterial bleeding	The goal of wound care is to stop bleeding, prevent infection, assess damage to underlying structures and promote healing. • Stop bleeding. [See SKILLS] • Clean wounds thoroughly with soap and clean water or antiseptic to remove any dirt, foreign bodies or dead/dying tissue. (Give local anaesthetic before cleaning the wound if available.) • Dress wounds with sterile gauze, if available. • Check perfusion beyond the wound (capillary refill and/or distal pulses) before and after dressing wounds. • Splint extremities with large lacerations to help with wound healing and pain control. [See SKILLS] • Stabilize but do not remove penetrating objects. • For snake bite, immobilize the extremity. [See WOUND MANAGEMENT in SKILLS] • For animal bites, consult advanced provider to assess for risk of infection and rabies exposure. Depending on vaccination status, management can be extremely time-sensitive. • Give tetanus vaccination if needed.

REMEMBER... Always assess, treat and monitor pain.

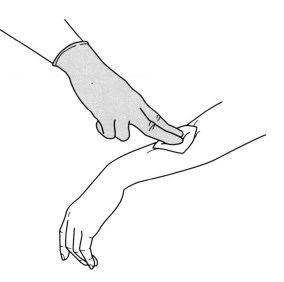

Applying direct pressure to a wound

SPECIAL CONSIDERATIONS

Management by injury mechanism

CONDITION	CONCERNING SIGNS AND SYMPTOMS	IN-DEPTH MANAGEMENT
Crush injury	• Fractures, bruising, soft tissue damage • Evidence of compartment syndrome (pain, firm muscle compartments, numbness, decreased pulses or pale skin) • Small amounts of red-brown urine	Crush injuries can have serious complications. Look for compartment syndrome (a build-up of pressure within the muscle compartments that can limit blood supply to muscles and nerves) and kidney damage due to by-products of muscle injury. • It is important to monitor urine output and look for red-brown urine (a concern for possible kidney damage). • Give IV fluids to help the kidneys maintain urine output. • Splint fractures to keep bone ends from causing further damage. • Plan for early surgical referral to release the pressure if compartment syndrome develops. • Patients may have many systemic problems related to muscle damage and should always be handed over to an advanced provider.
Blast injury	• Injury to air-filled organs (such as lung, stomach and bowel) • Delayed symptoms of tachypnoea, hypoxia, chest pain, cough with or without blood • Abdominal pain, nausea, vomiting with or without blood • Tympanic membrane (ear drum) rupture: hearing loss, ringing in the ears, pain, ear bleeding • Other injuries, burns, exposure to chemicals or toxins	An explosive blast can cause injuries in three ways: 1. Visible injuries from shrapnel (fragments of metal released by an explosive device) or burns from heat or chemicals released; 2. Internal (often hidden) injuries from the change in pressure caused by the blast. The stomach and bowel, lungs, and ears are commonly injured; and 3. Additional blunt injuries that result when the body is thrown by the blast. • Examine carefully for pneumothorax. • Give oxygen if there is difficulty in breathing. [See SKILLS] • Update tetanus. • Burns should be dressed and fluid needs calculated based on burn area. [See SKILLS] • If the patient has abdominal pain, consider bowel perforation, give IV fluids [See SKILLS] • Prepare for rapid surgical referral.

INTRO

ABCDE

TRAUMA

BREATHING

SHOCK

AMS

SKILLS

GLOSSARY

REFS & QUICK CARDS

Management by injury mechanism

CONDITION	CONCERNING SIGNS AND SYMPTOMS	IN-DEPTH MANAGEMENT
Burn injury	• Skin colour can range from pink, red, pale, or black, depending on the burn depth. The burn may or may not have blisters. • The following may suggest inhalation or airway injury. – Soot (ash) around nose or mouth, or singed (burned) nasal hairs – Swelling to lips or mouth – Voice changes	Burns can affect the whole body and cause soft tissue injury, swelling and shock resulting from fluid loss due to the burn. The goal of burn management is to stop the burning process, watch for swelling and compensate for fluid loss. In significant burn injury, fluid leaks into the skin and surrounding tissue causing swelling and shock. • Burns involving the airway can rapidly cause airway obstruction. • It is crucial to replace fluid loss and anticipate ongoing losses. – In order to calculate the IV fluid requirements, it is important to determine the depth of the burn and the percentage of body surface area (BSA) that is burned. [See SKILLS] • Do not forget to give tetanus vaccination and pain relief for burn injuries. • Remove all jewelry and elevate the burned limb if possible. • Burns are at high risk for infection, even with good care. Clean and dress the wound carefully. [See SKILLS] **BURNS REQUIRING RAPID HANDOVER/TRANSFER:** • Serious burns to >15% of body [See SKILLS] • Burns involving the hands, face, groin area, joints, or circumferential burns • Inhalation injury • Burns with other associated trauma • Any burn in very young or elderly people • Significant pre-burn illness (such as diabetes)

Workbook question 5: Approach to Trauma

Using the workbook section above, list what you would DO to manage the following injuries.

INJURY	MANAGEMENT
Pelvic fracture	1. _____
	2. _____
	3. _____
	4. _____
Burn injury in an adult	1. _____
	2. _____
	3. _____
	4. _____
Abdominal injury	1. _____
	2. _____
	3. _____
	4. _____

INTRO

ABCDE

TRAUMA

BREATHING

SHOCK

AMS

SKILLS

GLOSSARY

REFS & QUICK CARDS

SPECIAL POPULATIONS

TRAUMA IN PREGNANCY

Any female patient aged 10–50 years should have a pregnancy test. Pregnancy causes many changes in physiology and there are added considerations for fetal well-being. Even minor trauma may cause harm to the mother and fetus. Women suffering trauma in the third trimester are at risk for placental abruption (where the placenta can separate from the uterus wall, resulting in bleeding), uterine rupture, and premature labour. Remember resuscitation of the mother resuscitates the fetus.

KEY ELEMENTS OF PATIENT HISTORY

- Gestational age (age of the fetus or number of weeks since last menstrual period).
- Any pregnancy complications.

PRIMARY SURVEY

- Airway: swelling in pregnancy can make airway obstruction more likely, so monitor closely.
- Breathing: the diaphragm is pushed up by the pregnant uterus, leaving less lung space for breathing.
- Circulation: check for vaginal bleeding; a pregnant uterus can also compress large blood vessels, causing hypotension. Place on left side with cervical spine precautions. [See SKILLS]
- Disability: always consider eclampsia if seizures/convulsions occur.
- Exposure: keep patient warm.

COMMON CONDITIONS CAUSED BY TRAUMA

- Preterm (early) labour with or without premature rupture of membranes (loss of the fluid surrounding the baby).
- Placental abruption or uterine rupture: causing blood loss and shock.
- Seizures/convulsions.

SPECIAL MANAGEMENT CONSIDERATIONS

- Plan early for handover/transfer to a specialist unit with obstetric care.
- If the uterus can be felt at the level of the umbilicus (belly button), this generally indicates that the patient is at least 20 weeks pregnant.
- If the woman is more than 20 weeks (5 months) pregnant, the pregnant uterus can compress the inferior vena cava, the large vessel that brings blood back to her heart, and can cause shock. When lying the pregnant patient flat, always place on the left side (on a spine board if immobilization necessary). [See SKILLS]
- Trauma in late pregnancy may trigger early labour. Prepare for neonatal resuscitation as well when trauma occurs in late pregnancy.

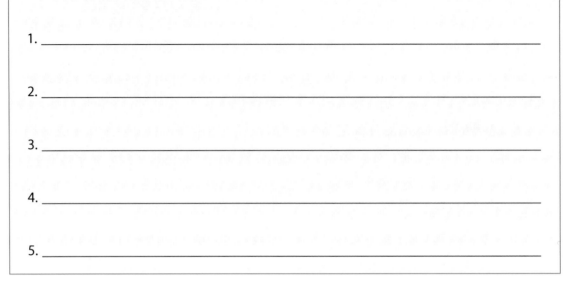

Workbook question 6: Approach to Trauma

Using the workbook section above, list the common conditions in a pregnant woman that can be caused by trauma.

1. _____

2. _____

3. _____

4. _____

5. _____

SPECIAL CONSIDERATIONS IN CHILDREN

67

Children can appear well after an injury, and yet deteriorate quickly. They have different injury patterns, and serious internal organ injuries may occur without overlying skull or rib fractures (paediatric bones are more flexible). Common management problems include over- or under-resuscitation, medication errors and failure to recognize hypothermia and hypoglycaemia.

Below are special considerations for injured children. Refer also to the ABCDE module for normal paediatric vital signs and additional details.

AIRWAY

- When neck trauma or cervical spine injury is suspected, use jaw thrust to manually open airway while maintaining cervical spine immobilization. Children have big heads and large tongues that may easily obstruct their airways. Young children and infants may require a pad under the shoulders to align the airway. [See SKILLS]

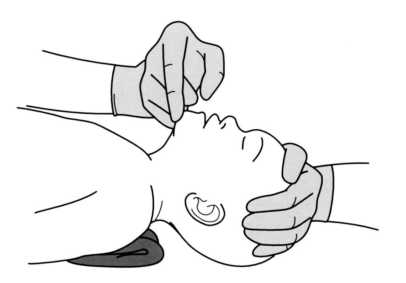

BREATHING

- If the child is not breathing adequately after opening the airway, assist breathing with a bag-valve-mask, ideally with oxygen.

- Give a breath every 4 seconds (15 breaths per minute) for older children and a breath every 3 seconds (20 breaths per minute) for infants. [See SKILLS]

INTRO

ABCDE

TRAUMA

BREATHING

SHOCK

AMS

SKILLS

GLOSSARY

REFS & QUICK CARDS

CIRCULATION

- For ongoing blood loss or evidence of poor perfusion in children with **normal nutritional status** (see also SKILLS):
  - place IV;
  - give IV fluids and re-assess. [See SKILLS]
- For **malnourished** children, fluids MUST be adjusted. [See SKILLS]
- For severe burn injury, initial bolus is with dextrose-containing fluids. [See SKILLS]
- If significant haemorrhage, arrange for blood transfusion or rapid handover/transfer to a centre capable of blood transfusion.

Location of brachial pulse in a child

DISABILITY

- Monitor child's level of consciousness with the **AVPU** scale (**A**lert, responsive to **V**erbal stimuli, responsive to **P**ainful stimuli, **U**nresponsive). AVPU is preferred to GCS in young children.
- Assess for and manage seizures/convulsions.
- Assess for and manage hypoglycaemia.

EXPOSURE

- Expose the entire body but watch for hypothermia.
- Protect the child's modesty at all times.
- Use log-roll to assess remainder of child's back and head.

Estimate weight in children based on age
Weight in kilograms = [age in years + 4] × 2
or use weight-estimation tools such as PAWPER tape, Mercy TAPE, or Broselow tape, etc.

GENERAL

Young children may be less able than adults to report events, even major events like being hit by a vehicle. Always consider the possibility of unwitnessed trauma in young children.

HEAD INJURIES

Head injuries are a common cause of death in children, and children frequently suffer from acute brain swelling after a severe head injury. If a paediatric patient has signs of traumatic brain injury, transport urgently to a facility with critical care and/or surgical capacity.

CHEST INJURIES

Chest injuries can be life-threatening, and children require less force for more serious internal injuries. The ribs are more flexible than in adults, and there may be extensive chest injuries without rib fractures.

ABDOMINAL INJURIES

Children's abdomens are relatively larger than adults, and the abdomen is a common site of injury in children. Injuries to the spleen and liver are especially common. Abdominal injuries should be considered in all paediatric trauma patients as they can be life-threatening and can cause severe internal bleeding.

BURN INJURIES

Burns in children can be difficult to manage. They require careful fluid resuscitation, close observation for airway swelling, and pain medications for dressing changes. In children who are burned, plan for rapid handover/transfer to a burn unit.

Workbook question 7: Approach to Trauma

Using the workbook section above, list the circulation considerations in children who suffer trauma.

1. _____

2. _____

3. _____

List the disability considerations in children who suffer trauma.

1. _____

2. _____

3. _____

DISPOSITION CONSIDERATIONS

Trauma patients can have complex injuries that may be hidden, and can worsen and die very quickly. Always refer seriously injured patients to a higher level of care for specialized treatment.

The following high-risk conditions always require handover/transfer to a specialist unit for ongoing care:

- Airway problem requiring intervention.
- Signs of shock:
    - Tension pneumothorax: perform needle decompression prior to transfer (will need urgent chest tube placement).
    - Pericardial tamponade: ensure IV fluids started and continued on transfer.
- Altered mental status (drowsy, lethargic, confused or unconscious).
- Trauma in pregnancy: place on left side for transport (needs specialist obstetric care).
- Child with ABCDE problem, burn, or any head, chest or abdominal injury.
- Any serious burn injury: assess the burn depth and total burn surface area, commence fluid resuscitation (transfer preferably to a specialist burns unit). [See SKILLS]

Other considerations for transfer:

- If a patient has required oxygen, arrange to continue it during transport and after handover.
- If an injured person is displaying signs of shock, ensure IV fluid started and continued during transfer. Ensure any external bleeding is controlled and monitored during transport.

INTRO

ABCDE

TRAUMA

BREATHING

SHOCK

AMS

SKILLS

GLOSSARY

REFS & QUICK CARDS

FACILITATOR-LED CASE SCENARIOS

These case scenarios will be presented in small groups. The following cases WILL NOT be assessed and are for practice only. It is important that you practise these scenarios as you will be assessed on how you lead a case in the following modules. For each case scenario the group must identify the critical findings and management needed and formulate a one-line summary for handover, including assessment findings and interventions. You should use the Quick Cards for these scenarios.

CASE #1: ADULT TRAUMA

A taxi driver brings in a man that was severely injured. You come outside to find a 30-year-old male lying in the back seat of the taxi in severe pain. He was in a car crash a few kilometers away. His jeans are soaked with blood, with bone sticking out of the right thigh.

1. What do you need to do in your initial approach?

2. Use the primary survey to assess and manage this patient. Ask the facilitator about look, listen and feel findings; use the Quick Card for reference as needed.

	ASSESSMENT	FINDINGS	INTERVENTION NEEDED?		INTERVENTIONS TO PERFORM:
AIRWAY			YES	NO	
BREATHING			YES	NO	
CIRCULATION			YES	NO	
DISABILITY			YES	NO	
EXPOSURE			YES	NO	

3. Formulate a short summary of this patient for handover.

CASE #2: PAEDIATRIC TRAUMA

A 5-year-old boy pulled a pan of boiling water off the stove at 8pm tonight. The boiling water spilled on him, burning his right side. His mother used a container of cool water to wash him down and then brought him in for evaluation. The child is crying and tells you he is in pain. He has burns to his right palm, and right inner arm up to the elbow, and the front of his chest and abdomen and the front of his right thigh. The mother does not know how much the child weighs.

1. What do you need to do in your initial approach?

2. Use the primary survey to assess and manage this patient. Ask the facilitator about look, listen and feel findings; use the Quick Card for reference as needed. Use the table below for your notes.

	ASSESSMENT	FINDINGS	INTERVENTION NEEDED?		INTERVENTIONS TO PERFORM:
AIRWAY			YES	NO	
BREATHING			YES	NO	
CIRCULATION			YES	NO	
DISABILITY			YES	NO	
EXPOSURE			YES	NO	

A. Calculate the total burn surface area in this child. Try to shade in the children's burn diagram for burn area estimation.

B. Explain how you will decide if this child needs IV fluids?

C. Calculate how much fluid is needed, explaining your method.

D. What fluid would you use?

3. Formulate a short summary of this patient for handover.

INTRO

ABCDE

TRAUMA

BREATHING

SHOCK

AMS

SKILLS

GLOSSARY

REFS & QUICK CARDS

MULTIPLE CHOICE QUESTIONS

Answer the questions below. Questions and answers will be discussed in the session.

1. Which of the following is a component of the trauma primary survey?

  A. Examine the arms for any fractures

  B. Check the skin color and temperature

  C. Examine the ears for any drainage of blood or clear liquid

  D. Check skin pinch

2. You are assessing a man who was in a car crash. He is very confused, but the remainder of his primary survey is normal. How do you perform a SAMPLE history if the patient is too confused to answer your questions?

  A. You do not need to do a SAMPLE history in a trauma patient

  B. Ask the patient repeatedly until he is able to answer

  C. Ask bystanders or family member for the information

  D. Assume that there is no important information

3. A 23-year-old man is carried in after diving head first into a river. He is speaking and his airway is open but he cannot walk or move his arms or legs. What is the first thing you must do?

  A. Place an IV line

  B. Examine him for other injuries

  C. Immobilize the cervical spine

  D. Give him a tetanus vaccination

4. You are evaluating a 21-year-old male who was in a motorcycle crash. He was thrown from the motorcycle and suffered injuries to his face, chest and legs. When you compress his pelvis, he screams in pain. His vital signs are: blood pressure 90/40 mmHg, heart rate 120 bpm, respiratory rate 25/min. What should be your next step?

  A. Place in a pelvic binder

  B. Administer tetanus vaccine

  C. Provide antibiotics

  D. Clean the abrasions with soap and water

5. A young woman has been brought in after an explosion. She has an open airway, a respiratory rate of 30/min, heart rate 125 bpm, blood pressure of 85/50 mmHg, has moist pale skin and she complains of abdominal pain. She has small wounds to her skin but there is no obvious bleeding. What would you do to manage this patient?

  A. Place two large-bore cannulae and give 1 litre of fluid

  B. Offer her a drink of water

  C. Check her temperature

  D. Provide antibiotics

Notes

....

....

....

....

....

....

....

....

....

....

....

....

....

....

....

Module 3: Approach to difficulty in breathing

Objectives

On completing this module you should be able to:

1. recognize signs of difficulty in breathing (DIB);

2. list the high-risk causes of difficulty in breathing;

3. perform critical actions for high-risk causes of difficulty in breathing.

Essential skills

- Basic airway manoeuvres
- Basic airway device insertion
- Management of choking
- Oxygen administration
- Bag-valve-mask ventilation
- Needle decompression for tension pneumothorax
- Three-sided dressing for sucking chest wound

KEY TERMS

Write the definition using the Glossary at the back of the workbook.

Accessory muscle use:

_____

Anaemia:

_____

Asthma:

_____

Chronic obstructive pulmonary disease (COPD):

_____

Circumferential burns:

_____

Crepitus:

_____

INTRO

ABCDE

TRAUMA

BREATHING

SHOCK

AMS

SKILLS

GLOSSARY

REFS & QUICK CARDS

Cyanosis:

_____

Diabetic ketoacidosis (DKA):

_____

Diaphoresis:

_____

Difficulty in breathing (DIB):

_____

Disposition:

_____

Drowning:

_____

Haemothorax:

_____

Heart attack:

_____

Heart failure:

_____

Hives:

_____

Hyperventilation:

_____

Inflammation:

_____

Ischaemia:

_____

Large-bore IV:

_____

Needle decompression:

_____

Pericardial effusion:

_____

Pleural effusion:

_____

Pleuritic:

_____

Pneumonia:

_____

Pulmonary embolism:

_____

Stridor:

_____

Tachycardia:

_____

Tachypnoea:

_____

Tracheal shift:

_____

Tripod position:

_____

Wheezing:

_____

Overview

Difficulty in breathing (DIB) is a term used to describe a range of conditions from a feeling of shortness of breath to abnormal breathing movements, or any increased effort required to breathe. DIB can result from problems in the upper or lower airways, the lungs, the heart or the muscles used for breathing; or from conditions that may cause faster breathing (such as anaemia or chemical imbalance).

DIB can be caused by:

- upper or lower airway obstruction (blockage by an object; by spasm of the airways, such as with asthma; by swelling due to allergy; infection or injury);
- fluid in the airspaces of the lung (such as from pneumonia or pulmonary oedema);
- air or fluid outside the lung causing lung collapse or compression (such as pneumothorax or effusion);
- blood clots in the vessels supplying the lungs;
- any other cause of decreased oxygen carried in the blood (such as anaemia);
- conditions that increase respiratory rate such as toxic ingestion, chemical imbalance (for example in diabetic ketoacidosis) or anxiety.

> **The goal of INITIAL ASSESSMENT** is to identify reversible causes of difficulty in breathing, and to recognize conditions that require urgent intervention or rapid transfer.
>
> **The goal of ACUTE MANAGEMENT** is to ensure the airway stays open and breathing is adequate to deliver oxygen to the organs.

This module will guide you through:

- ABCDE key elements
- ASK: key history findings (SAMPLE history)
- CHECK: secondary exam findings
- Possible causes
- DO: management
- Special considerations in children
- Disposition considerations

REMEMBER...

- **ALWAYS START WITH THE ABCDE APPROACH**, intervening as needed.
- **Then** do a **SAMPLE history.**
- **Then** do a **secondary exam.**

ABCDE: KEY ELEMENTS FOR PATIENTS WITH DIFFICULTY IN BREATHING

For the patient with difficulty in breathing, the following are key elements that should be considered in the ABCDE approach.

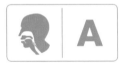

AIRWAY
A person with difficulty in breathing may have airway swelling caused by a **severe allergic reaction (anaphylaxis)** or **choking** (obstruction from a foreign body). Stridor suggests serious airway narrowing.

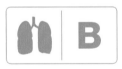

BREATHING
Hypotension with absent breath sounds on one side – especially with distended (swollen or enlarged) neck veins or tracheal shift – may indicate **tension pneumothorax.** Wheezing may indicate asthma or severe allergic reaction.

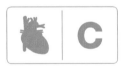

CIRCULATION
Shock, heart attack, heart failure and **severe infection** can all present with poor perfusion and difficulty in breathing. Poor perfusion sends signals to the brain to increase the rate of breathing, which can feel and look like difficulty in breathing. Check for signs of shock by checking capillary refill, heart rate and blood pressure. Swelling in the legs or crackles in the lungs can indicate **heart failure** and **fluid overload** as a cause of difficulty in breathing.

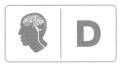

DISABILITY

Patients with decreased level of consciousness may not be able to protect their airways. **Drugs**, **infection** or **injury** can directly affect the part of the brain that controls breathing. Assess for paralyzing conditions affecting the breathing muscles.

Check level of consciousness with the AVPU scale:

A: **A**lert

V: Responds to **V**oice

P: Responds to **P**ain

U: **U**nresponsive

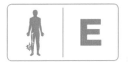

EXPOSURE

Expose the patient fully to assess for abnormal chest wall movement and any signs of trauma. **Penetrating trauma** to the back, chest, underarms or abdomen may cause lung injury and is often missed.

ASK: KEY HISTORY FINDINGS FOR PATIENTS WITH DIFFICULTY IN BREATHING

Use the SAMPLE approach to obtain a history from the patient and/or family.

If the history identifies an ABCDE condition, STOP AND RETURN IMMEDIATELY TO ABCDE to manage it.

S: SIGNS AND SYMPTOMS

- **When did the symptoms start and was onset sudden? Do they come and go and how long do they last? Have they changed over time and has there been a similar episode previously?**

  Sudden difficulty in breathing can suggest airway obstruction such as by a foreign body; swelling of the airway from allergic reaction or infection; trauma to the airway, lungs, heart or chest wall; or inhalation of hot gases or smoke. Acute heart problems such as heart attack, abnormal heart rhythm or valve problems can cause rapid onset DIB. A history of rapid or deep breathing may suggest poisoning, high acid levels in the blood (infection or diabetic ketoacidosis) or anxiety. DIB that starts slowly is more common with infection and chronic conditions such as a gradual build-up of fluid around the lungs (as occurs in TB and heart failure), fluid around the heart (from TB or kidney disease), lung cancer or diseases affecting the function of the chest wall. Recurrent difficulty in breathing associated with wheeze may suggest asthma or COPD.

- **Did anything trigger the difficulty in breathing and what makes it better or worse?**

  A history of allergies may suggest that the airway is blocked by swelling due to a severe allergic reaction. Inhaling smoke or hot gas (such as in fires) or some chemicals may cause

INTRO
ABCDE
TRAUMA
BREATHING
SHOCK
AMS
SKILLS
GLOSSARY
REFS & QUICK CARDS

DIB through upper airway injury and swelling. Exposure to some chemicals (such as certain pesticides) can cause fluid to build up in the airways and can cause weakness in the muscles involved in breathing. Difficulty in breathing that gets worse when the person lies flat can be due to fluid in the lungs.

- **Is there any tongue or lip swelling, or voice changes?**

  Swelling to the mouth, lips, tongue or upper throat, or a change in voice can suggest a severe allergic reaction or other inflammation of the airway.

- **Are there abnormal sounds with breathing?**

  High-pitched or 'squeaking' sounds when breathing IN may be stridor, which is caused by narrowing of the upper airway and may suggest severe allergic reaction or other airway obstruction. Wheezing – a high-pitched sound with breathing OUT – is caused by narrowing or spasm of the lower airways in the lungs and can suggest asthma, COPD, heart failure or allergic reactions. Gurgling sounds with breathing suggest that there is mucus, blood or other fluid in the airway.

- **Is there pain associated with the difficulty in breathing?**

  Difficulty in breathing with chest pain can suggest heart attack, pneumothorax, pneumonia or trauma to the lungs, ribs or ribcage muscles. In particular, pain that is worse with deep breaths (pleuritic pain) may suggest infection or blood clot in the lung (pulmonary embolism).

- **Is there fever or cough?**

  Fever suggests infection. Lung infection and any severe infection may cause fluid in the lungs. A cough may indicate fluid in the lungs from pneumonia or oedema. Cough and wheezing may suggest asthma or COPD.

- **Is there foot or leg swelling or recent pregnancy?**

  Difficulty in breathing with oedema of both feet or legs can suggest heart failure with fluid back-up to the lungs and body. Difficulty in breathing with swelling and pain in one leg may suggest a clot in a leg vein that has travelled to the lung (pulmonary embolism). Pregnancy is a risk factor for both pulmonary embolism and heart failure.

A: ALLERGIES

- **Any allergies to medications or other substances? Any recent insect bites or stings?**

  Severe allergic reactions may cause difficulty in breathing due to airway swelling. People can have severe allergic reactions to almost anything, but food, plants, medications and insect bites/stings are the most common.

M: MEDICATIONS

- **Currently taking any medications?**

  Ask about new medications and changes in doses. New medications can cause allergies with associated difficulty in breathing. Accidental overdose of some medications can stop or slow breathing.

INTRO

ABCDE

TRAUMA

BREATHING

SHOCK

AMS

SKILLS

GLOSSARY

REFS & QUICK CARDS

P: PAST MEDICAL HISTORY

- **Is there a history of asthma or chronic obstructive pulmonary disease (COPD)?**

  Asthma and COPD often cause episodes of difficulty in breathing. A history of prior hospitalization or intubation for these conditions suggests a high-risk patient.

- **Is there a history of heart disease or kidney disease?**

  People with a history of heart or kidney failure may have fluid in the lungs. Heart attack may present with difficulty in breathing.

- **Is there a history of tuberculosis (TB) or cancer?**

  Conditions such as tuberculosis and cancer can cause build up of fluid in the sac around the heart (pericardial effusion) or build-up of fluid outside the lung (pleural effusion), both of which can cause a feeling of difficulty in breathing.

- **Is there a history of diabetes?**

  Diabetes can cause diabetic crisis (diabetic ketoacidosis or DKA). DKA causes fast breathing that may be reported as difficulty in breathing.

- **Is there a history of smoking?**

  Smoking increases the risk of asthma, COPD, lung cancer and heart attack.

- **Is there a history of HIV?**

  HIV infection increases the risk of other infections.

L: LAST ORAL INTAKE

- **When did the person last eat or drink?**

  A full stomach puts the patient at risk of vomiting and possible choking.

E: EVENTS SURROUNDING ILLNESS

- **What was the person doing when the difficulty in breathing started?**

  Always consider choking if DIB started while eating or drinking. DIB with exercise might be due to heart attack, especially when there is also chest pain.

- **Was the patient found in or near water?**

  Always consider drowning (inhalation of water) in a person found in or near water. Even a small amount of inhaled water can cause serious lung damage, which can worsen over time.

- **Has there been exposure to pesticides or other chemicals?**

  Inhaled chemicals can cause DIB by irritating the airways and lungs. Some pesticides used in farming can be absorbed through the skin, causing fluid buildup in the airways and lungs. Exposure to gases from a fire is often associated with chemical inhalation.

- **Has there been any recent trauma?**

  DIB with trauma is concerning for rib fractures, pneumothorax, haemothorax, and heart or lung bruising.

Workbook question 1: Difficulty in breathing

Using the workbook section above, list five questions about past medical history you would ask when taking a SAMPLE history.

1. _____

2. _____

3. _____

4. _____

5. _____

CHECK: SECONDARY EXAMINATION FINDINGS FOR PATIENTS WITH DIFFICULTY IN BREATHING

DIB may present with changes in respiratory rate, respiratory effort, or low oxygen saturation. Always assess ABCDE first. The initial ABCDE approach identifies and manages life-threatening conditions. The secondary exam looks for changes in the patient's condition or less obvious causes which may have been missed during ABCDE. If the secondary examination identifies an ABCDE condition, **STOP AND RETURN IMMEDIATELY TO ABCDE to manage it.**

LOOK

Look for signs of respiratory failure:

- Accessory muscle use and increased work of breathing.
- Difficulty speaking in full sentences.
- Inability to lie down or lean back.
- Diaphoresis (excessive sweating) and mottled skin.
- Confusion, irritability, agitation.
- Poor chest wall movement.
- Cyanosis (blue skin colour, especially lips and fingertips).

Look at the pupils for size and reactivity:

- Very small pupils suggest possible opioid overdose or exposure to chemicals (including pesticides).
- Unequal or abnormally shaped pupils suggest head injury which can cause abnormal breathing.

Look at the face, nose and mouth:

- Cyanosis around the lips or nose suggests low oxygen levels in the blood.
- Pale inner surface of lower eyelids suggests severe anaemia.
- Swelling of the lips, tongue and mouth suggests an allergic reaction.
- Soot around the mouth or nose, burned facial hair or facial burns suggest smoke inhalation and airway burns.
- Bleeding or swelling of the airway may be due to trauma.

Look at the neck and chest:

- Distended neck veins can be due to a back-up of blood due to heart failure, tension pneumothorax or pericardial tamponade.
- Excessive muscle use in the neck and chest (between the ribs) suggests significant respiratory difficulty.
- If the trachea is shifted to one side, think about tension pneumothorax or tumour.
- Swelling or redness of the neck suggests infection or trauma.
- Examine the entire neck and chest carefully for bruising, wounds or other signs of trauma.

Look at the rate and pattern of breathing:

- People with wheeze may take longer to breathe out because of narrowing of the lower airways in the lung.
- Fast breathing can be due to dehydration, severe infection, chemical imbalance in the blood, poisoning or anxiety.
- Slow and shallow breathing might be due to opioid overdose. Look for very small pupils and altered mental status.
- Chest wall injury is often associated with pain that limits the ability to take deep breaths.
- A flail chest occurs when multiple rib fractures cause a segment of the rib cage to be separated from the rest of the chest wall. The segment may appear to be moving in the opposite direction from the rest of chest wall during breathing.

Look at the legs:

- Swelling to the both lower legs suggests heart failure as a cause of difficulty in breathing.
- Swelling to one leg may be due to a blood clot in the leg. If there is also difficulty in breathing, this may mean that part of the clot has traveled to the lung.

Look at the skin:

- Bites can be a source of allergic reaction.
- Rashes, such as hives, can indicate allergic reaction. When associated with difficulty in breathing, rashes can indicate widespread (systemic) infection.
- Pallor (pale skin) can indicate anaemia as a cause of DIB.
- Circumferential burns (a burn that goes entirely around a body part) to the chest can restrict chest wall expansion and limit breathing.

LISTEN

Listen to the breath sounds:

- Stridor suggests partial upper airway obstruction, which may be due to a foreign object, mass, or swelling from trauma or infection.

- Decreased or absent breath sounds suggest abnormal air movement in the lungs. This can be due to air or fluid around the lung (pneumothorax, haemothorax, effusion), narrowing or foreign body blockage of the airways, and infection or tumour in or around the lung.

- Wheezing, in particular, suggests lower airway obstruction such as from asthma, COPD, allergic reaction, foreign body or tumour.

- Crackles or crepitations suggest fluid in the airspaces of the lung.

Listen to the heart sounds:

- Abnormal heart rhythms can cause the heart to pump blood abnormally, leading to poor perfusion and a feeling of difficulty in breathing.

- Difficulty in breathing accompanied by heart murmurs can suggest damage to the heart valves.

- Muffled or distant heart sounds accompanying low blood pressure, fast heart rate and distended neck veins suggest pericardial tamponade.

FEEL

Feel the ribs and chest wall:

- Deformities and abnormal movement when pressing on the chest wall suggest rib fracture.

- Crepitus (crackling or popping when pressing on the skin of the chest wall) may suggest underlying fracture or air under the skin (associated with pneumothorax).

- Unequal expansion of the chest wall suggests pneumothorax, haemothorax, or flail chest.

Percuss the chest wall [See SKILLS]:

- Hollow sounds (hyperresonance) on one side when tapping the chest wall suggest pneumothorax.

- Dull sounds when tapping the chest wall may indicate fluid or blood either inside the airspaces of the lungs or between the lungs and the chest wall.

INTRO
ABCDE
TRAUMA
BREATHING
SHOCK
AMS
SKILLS
GLOSSARY
REFS & QUICK CARDS

Workbook question 2: Difficulty in breathing

Using the workbook section above, list three signs you should LOOK for in a patient with difficulty in breathing.

1. _____

2. _____

3. _____

List four things you should LISTEN for in a patient with difficulty in breathing.

1. _____

2. _____

3. _____

4. _____

List three things you should FEEL the chest wall for in a patient with difficulty in breathing.

1. _____

2. _____

3. _____

POSSIBLE CAUSES OF DIFFICULTY IN BREATHING

The causes of difficulty in breathing can be organized by body area: airway, lung, heart, or whole body.

Key airway causes	
CONDITION	SIGNS AND SYMPTOMS
Foreign body in the airway	• Acute difficulty in breathing • Visible secretions, vomit or foreign body in the airway • Abnormal sounds from the airway (such as stridor, snoring, gurgling) • Coughing • Drooling
Severe allergic reaction	• Swelling of lips, tongue and mouth • Stridor and/or wheezing • Rash or hives • May have tachycardia and hypotension • Exposure to known allergen

CONDITION	SIGNS AND SYMPTOMS
Airway swelling (due to inflammation/ infection)	• Stridor • Hoarse voice • Drooling or difficulty swallowing (indicates severe swelling) • Unable to lie down • May have fever (with infection)
Airway burns	• History of exposure to chemical or fire • Burns to head and neck (or singed facial hair or soot around nose or mouth) • Stridor • Change in voice

Key lung causes

CONDITION	SIGNS AND SYMPTOMS
Pneumonia	• Fever and cough • Gradually more laboured breathing • Pain worse with breathing (pleuritic) • Abnormal lung examination (crackles)
Asthma/COPD	• Wheezing • Cough • Accessory muscle use • Tripod position (see figure) • May have history of smoking or allergies
Pneumothorax	• Decreased breath sounds on one side • Sudden onset • Hollow sounds (hyperresonance) to percussion on affected side [See SKILLS] • May have pain that worsens with breathing • May have history of trauma or evidence of rib fracture • Hypotension with distended neck veins and decreased breath sounds on one side indicate tension pneumothorax.
Haemothorax	• Decreased breath sounds on affected side • Dull sounds with percussion [See SKILLS] • May have a history of trauma, cancer or tuberculosis Shock (if large haemothorax)
Pleural effusion	• Decreased breath sounds on one or both sides • Dull sounds with percussion [See SKILLS] • May have history of cancer, tuberculosis, heart disease or kidney disease • Acute or chronic difficulty in breathing
Acute chest syndrome in a patient with sickle dell disease	• History of sickle cell disease • Chest pain • Fever • Hypoxia

INTRO

ABCDE

TRAUMA

BREATHING

SHOCK

AMS

SKILLS

GLOSSARY

REFS & QUICK CARDS

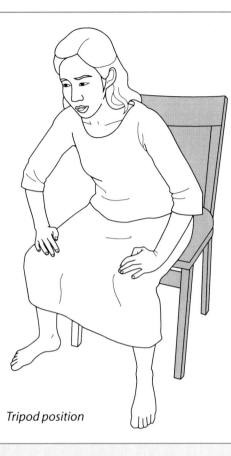

Tripod position

Key heart causes

CONDITION	SIGNS AND SYMPTOMS
Heart attack	• Pressure, tightness or crushing feeling in the chest • Diaphoresis and mottled skin • Nausea or vomiting • Signs of heart failure • History of smoking, heart disease, hypertension, diabetes, high cholesterol, family history of heart problems
Heart failure	• Worse with exertion • Worse when lying flat • Swelling to both legs • Distended neck veins • Crackles may be heard in the lungs • May have chest pain
Pericardial tamponade	• Signs of poor perfusion (tachycardia, tachypnoea, hypotension, pale skin, cold extremities, capillary refill greater than 3 seconds) • Distended neck veins • Muffled heart sounds • May have dizziness, confusion, altered mental status • History of tuberculosis, trauma, malignancy, kidney failure

Key systemic causes

CONDITION	SIGNS AND SYMPTOMS
Anaemia	• Pale skin and inner lower eyelids • Tachycardia • Tachypnoea • History of haemorrhage, malnourishment, cancer, pregnancy, malaria, sickle cell disease, renal failure
Opioid overdose	• Clinical or recreational opioid use • Altered mental status • Very small pupils • Slow, shallow breathing
Diabetic ketoacidosis	• May have known history of diabetes • Deep or rapid breathing • Frequent urination • Sweet smelling breath • High glucose in blood or urine • Dehydrated

Workbook question 3: Difficulty in breathing

Using the workbook section above, list the possible cause of difficulty in breathing next to the history and physical findings below.

HISTORY AND PHYSICAL FINDINGS	LIKELY CAUSE
A 20-year-old man presents with difficulty in breathing, wheezing and: • swelling of lips, tongue and mouth • rash or hives (patches of pale or red, itchy, warm, swollen skin) • tachycardia and hypotension • history of allergies • exposure to known allergen	
A 50-year-old woman presents with difficulty in breathing, signs of poor perfusion (tachycardia, tachypnoea, hypotension, pale skin, cold extremities, capillary refill >3 seconds) and: • distended neck veins • muffled heart sounds • history of tuberculosis	

INTRO

ABCDE

TRAUMA

BREATHING

SHOCK

AMS

SKILLS

GLOSSARY

REFS & QUICK CARDS

DO: MANAGEMENT

FIRST PERFORM ABCDE ASSESSMENT AND INTERVENE FOR LIFE-THREATENING CONDITIONS.

Assess and manage airway and provide bag-mask-ventilation (BVM) for any patient who is not breathing or not breathing adequately (too slow for age or too shallow); any unconscious patient with abnormal (slow, shallow, gasping or noisy) breathing; or any patient with a pulse who is not breathing. For patients without a pulse, follow relevant CPR protocols.

CONDITION	MANAGEMENT CONSIDERATIONS
Airway inflammation or burns	Keep patients calm. Give oxygen if you can do this without upsetting the patient. [See SKILLS]
	If the patient is fully alert and no spinal injury suspected, the seated position may be more comfortable.
	Patients with airway burns may require early intubation as the airway can swell and block quickly; delays may make intubation more difficult.
	A person with airway inflammation or burns requires urgent handover/transfer.
Choking	Use age-appropriate chest thrusts/abdominal thrusts/back blows. [See SKILLS]
Allergic reaction	Remove the allergen, if possible. For severe allergic reaction with difficulty breathing give intramuscular adrenaline as soon as possible. Give oxygen for severe cases. [See SKILLS]
Asthma/COPD	Administer salbutamol as soon as possible. Give oxygen if indicated. [See SKILLS]
Fever	Give antibiotics as soon as possible if infection might be the cause of difficulty in breathing. If the patient has signs of poor perfusion, give IV fluids with caution to avoid fluid overload. [See SKILLS]
Heart attack	Give aspirin. While oxygen is no longer recommended in all patients with heart attack, it should initially be given to patients with shock or difficulty in breathing. [See SKILLS] For those patients who already have nitroglycerin, you can assist them in taking it if perfusion is adequate.
Chronic, severe anaemia	Give IV fluids more slowly and check the lungs for crackles (fluid overload) frequently. [See SKILLS] These patients may need handover/transfer for blood transfusion.
Diabetic ketoacidosis	Give IV fluids. [See SKILLS] A person with diabetic ketoacidosis is extremely ill and requires urgent transfer to an advanced provider.
Opioid overdose	Support breathing with a bag-valve-mask as needed. Give naloxone. [See SKILLS]
Pleural effusion or haemothorax	Give oxygen. [See SKILLS] Arrange for handover/transfer immediately. Many of these patients will need a chest tube or other drainage.
Trauma	All trauma patients with difficulty in breathing should be given oxygen. IV fluid should be given to help fill the heart if either pericardial tamponade or tension pneumothorax is suspected. Needle decompression should be performed if tension pneumothorax is suspected. Treat sucking chest wounds with a 3-sided dressing. [See SKILLS] The patient will need urgent handover/transfer for a chest tube if needle decompression is performed or a 3-sided dressing is applied.
Acute chest syndrome	Give oxygen, IV fluids, antibiotics. May need transfer for advanced management.

Workbook question 4: Difficulty in breathing

Using the workbook section above, list what you would DO to manage a person who presents with:

DIB, coughing. You suspect choking.

1. _____
2. _____

DIB, high fever, cough. You suspect serious infection.

1. _____
2. _____

DIB, hoarse voice and stridor on breathing in. You to suspect airway inflammation.

1. _____
2. _____
3. _____

SPECIAL CONSIDERATIONS IN CHILDREN

The following are *danger signs* in children:

- Signs of airway obstruction (unable to swallow saliva/drooling or stridor).
- Increased breathing effort (fast breathing, nasal flaring, grunting, chest indrawing or retractions).
- Cyanosis (blue colour of the skin, especially at the lips and fingertips).
- Altered mental status (lethargy or unusual sleepiness, agitation).
- Poor feeding or drinking.
- Vomiting everything.
- Seizures/convulsions.
- Low temperature (hypothermia).

REMEMBER...

- Wheezing in children can be caused by viral infection, asthma or an inhaled object blocking the airway.
- Stridor in children can be caused by an object stuck in the upper airway OR airway swelling.
- Children may present with rapid breathing as the only sign of pneumonia.
- Rapid breathing can also indicate diabetic crisis (DKA), which may be the first sign of diabetes in a child.

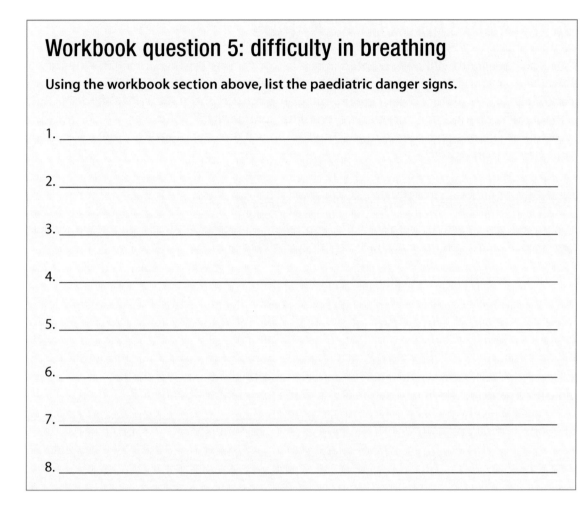

Workbook question 5: difficulty in breathing

Using the workbook section above, list the paediatric danger signs.

1. _____

2. _____

3. _____

4. _____

5. _____

6. _____

7. _____

8. _____

DISPOSITION CONSIDERATIONS

- Keep in mind that the effects of inhaled medications such as salbutamol last for only approximately 3 hours. Patients need to be monitored closely.

- If a patient with a severe allergic reaction is given adrenaline, the reaction can return when the adrenaline wears off. Patients need to be monitored closely.

- Naloxone only lasts about 1 hour. Most opioid medications last longer than this, so patients may need repeat naloxone doses.

- Following immersion in water (drowning), a person may develop late signs of breathing problems after several hours and should be observed closely.

- Never leave patients who might need definitive airway placement unmonitored during handover/transfer. Ensure that a new provider is monitoring the patient before leaving.

- Make transfer arrangements as early as possible for any patient who may require assisted ventilation.

INTRO
ABCDE
TRAUMA
BREATHING
SHOCK
AMS
SKILLS
GLOSSARY
REFS & QUICK CARDS

FACILITATOR-LED CASE SCENARIOS

These case scenarios will be presented in small groups. One participant will be identified as the lead and will be assessed while the rest of the group writes the responses in the workbook. To complete a case scenario, the group must identify the critical findings and management needed and formulate a one-line summary for handover, which includes assessment findings and interventions. You should use the Quick Cards for these scenarios while being assessed.

CASE #1: ADULT WITH DIFFICULTY IN BREATHING

A 22-year-old man arrives by taxi. He was robbed on the street, and was stabbed in the left chest with a knife. He is now having severe difficulty in breathing.

1. What do you need to do in your initial approach?

2. Use the ABCDE approach to assess and manage this patient. Ask the facilitator about look, listen and feel findings; use the Quick Cards for reference as needed.

	ASSESSMENT FINDINGS	INTERVENTION NEEDED?		INTERVENTIONS TO PERFORM:
AIRWAY		YES	NO	
BREATHING		YES	NO	
CIRCULATION		YES	NO	
DISABILITY		YES	NO	
EXPOSURE		YES	NO	

3. Formulate one sentence to summarize this patient for handover.

CASE #2: PAEDIATRIC PATIENT WITH DIFFICULTY IN BREATHING

A mother brings in her 6-year-old son for difficulty in breathing. The mother states that her son has been having difficulty breathing for the past 3 days. She says he makes funny noises when he breathes.

1. What do you need to do in your initial approach?

2. Use the ABCDE approach to assess and manage this patient. Ask the facilitator about look, listen and feel findings; use the Quick Card for reference as needed.

	ASSESSMENT	FINDINGS	INTERVENTION NEEDED?		INTERVENTIONS TO PERFORM:
AIRWAY			YES	NO	
BREATHING			YES	NO	
CIRCULATION			YES	NO	
DISABILITY			YES	NO	
EXPOSURE			YES	NO	

3. Formulate one sentence to summarize this patient for handover.

INTRO

ABCDE

TRAUMA

BREATHING

SHOCK

AMS

SKILLS

GLOSSARY

REFS & QUICK CARDS

MULTIPLE CHOICE QUESTIONS

Answer the questions below. Questions and answers will be discussed in the session

1. You are evaluating a 34-year-old female complaining of difficulty in breathing, coughing, and fever for 3 days. Which of the following actions should you do first?

   A. Check blood pressure

   B. Administer antibiotics

   C. Start an IV

   D. Check the lung sounds

2. A 67-year-old man with a history of a heart attack is complaining of difficulty in breathing that is worse whenever he lies flat. His legs are both swollen, which has become worse in the past 2 weeks. What is the most likely cause of his difficulty in breathing?

   A. Heart failure

   B. Asthma

   C. Pneumothorax

   D. Pneumonia

3. There was a fire in a nearby house and a patient is brought to you with burned nasal hairs and shortness of breath. What should you do first?

   A. Give oxygen

   B. Give intramuscular adrenaline

   C. Start an IV line

   D. Perform needle decompression

4. A 30-year-old woman was stung by a bee and now has difficulty in breathing, facial swelling, and a rash. She has a history of severe allergic reactions to bee stings. What medication should you give her?

   A. Naloxone

   B. Benzodiazepine

   C. Adrenaline

   D. Aspirin

5. You are assessing a 10-year-old boy for difficulty in breathing. You notice that the skin on his fingertips and around his mouth has a blue color. What is this finding called?

   A. Retractions

   B. Nasal flaring

   C. Crepitus

   D. Cyanosis

Module 4: Approach to shock

Objectives

On completing this module you should be able to:

1. recognize signs of shock/poor perfusion;

2. perform critical actions for patients with shock;

3. assess fluid status;

4. select appropriate fluid administration based on patient age, weight and condition;

5. recognize malnourishment, anaemia and burns and adjust fluid resuscitation.

Essential skills

- Oxygen administration
- IV line placement
- Fluid status assessment
- IV fluid resuscitation
- Burn management
- Needle decompression
- Three-sided dressing
- Direct pressure for bleeding control
- Uterine massage for bleeding control
- Trauma secondary survey

KEY TERMS

Write the definition using the Glossary at the back of the workbook.

Bolus:

_____

Bradycardia:

_____

Capillary refill:

_____

Cholera:

_____

INTRO

ABCDE

TRAUMA

BREATHING

SHOCK

AMS

SKILLS

GLOSSARY

REFS & QUICK CARDS

Diaphoresis:

_____

Dehydration:

_____

Diabetic ketoacidosis (DKA):

_____

Dilation (of blood vessels):

_____

Disposition:

_____

Ectopic pregnancy:

_____

Fluid status:

_____

Fontanelle:

_____

Gastroenteritis:

_____

Large-bore IV:

_____

Lethargy:

_____

Oral rehydration solution (ORS):

_____

Perfusion:

_____

Pericardial tamponade:

_____

Resuscitation:

_____

Shock:

_____

Skin pinch testing:

_____

Overview

Poor perfusion is when the body is not able to get enough oxygen-carrying blood to vital organs. When organ function is affected, this is called shock and can lead rapidly to death. Infants, children and older adults are more likely to be affected by shock.

Causes of poor perfusion which may lead to shock include:

- loss of blood (haemorrhage);

- loss of fluid due to diarrhoea, vomiting, extensive burns or excess urination (such as caused by high blood sugar);

- poor fluid intake. Small children, the elderly and the very ill may be unable to drink enough fluids without assistance and are at risk of dehydration;

- abnormal relaxation and enlargement (dilation) of the blood vessels (with the same amount of blood inside the vessel) can lower blood pressure. This can occur in severe infection, spinal cord injury and severe allergic reaction;

- poor filling of the heart can result from blood or other fluid in the sac around the heart (pericardial tamponade), or increased pressure in the chest that can shift and block the vessels returning blood to the heart (tension pneumothorax);

- failure of the heart muscle to pump effectively can be due to a heart attack (vessel blockage that causes acute heart muscle damage); inflammation or other disease of the heart muscle itself; an abnormal rhythm or valve problems. (Shock due to failure of the heart to pump effectively is sometimes called cardiogenic shock.)

> **The goal of INITIAL ASSESSMENT** is to identify shock and any reversible causes of shock.
>
> **The goal of ACUTE MANAGEMENT** is to restore perfusion (oxygen delivery to the organs) and address ongoing fluid loss where possible.

This module will guide you through:

- ABCDE key elements
- ASK: key history findings (SAMPLE history)
- CHECK: secondary examination findings
- Possible causes
- DO: management
- Special considerations in children
- Disposition considerations

REMEMBER...

- **ALWAYS START WITH THE ABCDE APPROACH,** intervening as needed.
- **Then do a SAMPLE history.**
- **Then do a secondary examination.**

ABCDE: KEY ELEMENTS IN SHOCK

For the person in shock, the following are key elements that should be considered in the ABCDE approach.

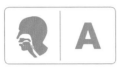

AIRWAY

Face/mouth swelling or voice changes can indicate an allergic reaction. A **severe allergic reaction** can cause shock.

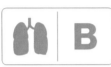

BREATHING

Wheezing can indicate a **severe allergic reaction** which can cause shock. Shock, difficulty in breathing and absent breath sounds on one side can indicate a **tension pneumothorax**. Poor perfusion itself can sometimes cause rapid breathing when vital organs do not receive enough oxygen. Severe **heart failure** can cause poor perfusion with difficulty in breathing when fluid backs up into the lungs. Any **infection** severe enough to cause shock may be associated with lung inflammation that causes difficulty in breathing.

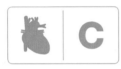

CIRCULATION

Shock can be caused by many types of **bleeding** (from the stomach or intestines, pregnancy-related, and internal and external **haemorrhage** from trauma). Shock can also result from the **fluid loss** associated with diarrhoea, vomiting, extensive burns, or excess urination (such as caused by high blood sugar).

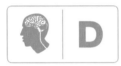

DISABILITY

Confusion in a person with poor perfusion suggests severe shock. Paralysis may indicate a **spinal cord injury** causing shock.

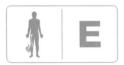

EXPOSURE

Look for signs of bleeding, trauma, and excessive sweating (diaphoresis). Hives can indicate allergic reaction, and other rashes can indicate systemic infection.

ASK: KEY HISTORY FINDINGS IN SHOCK

Use the SAMPLE approach to obtain a history from the patient and/or family.

If the history identifies an ABCDE condition, STOP AND RETURN IMMEDIATELY TO ABCDE to manage it.

S: SIGNS AND SYMPTOMS

- **Has there been vomiting and/or diarrhoea? For how long?**

  Fluid losses through vomiting and diarrhoea can be severe and can lead to shock. The amount of vomiting or diarrhoea can help give a rough estimate of the risk for shock, so always ask about frequency of episodes.

- **Has the person had blood in stool or vomit?**

  Bleeding in the stomach and/or intestines can be severe before it is recognized. A person can lose a significant portion of his or her blood volume in the intestines. Blood may appear black in both vomit and stools.

- **Has there been any vaginal bleeding?**

  Vaginal bleeding may be related to pregnancy in women of childbearing years. Always ask about pregnancy status, last menstrual period, any missed periods, or known recent pregnancy. Blood loss from normal delivery or miscarriage can cause shock. A pregnancy developing outside the uterus (ectopic pregnancy) can also be life-threatening if it ruptures. Ectopic pregnancy rupture can occur before a woman even knows she is pregnant. Other causes of vaginal bleeding are masses in the cervix or uterus.

- **Has the person had any chest pain?**

  Chest pain may suggest the person has had a heart attack. The muscle damage to the heart from a heart attack can reduce its ability to pump blood around the body, which can cause shock.

- **Has there been fever?**

  Fever may suggest infection as the cause of shock. Severe infection causes both dilation of the blood vessels (which lowers blood pressure) and fluid leakage from the blood vessels (with fluid loss into the tissues).

- **Has there been any exposure to toxins, medications, insect stings or other substances?**

  Severe allergic reactions can lead to shock. Additionally, many medications, including blood pressure and seizure/convulsion medications, can cause shock.

- **Has there been altered mental status or unusual sleepiness?**

  The brain is one of the last organs to be affected by poor perfusion, so altered mental status may be a sign of severe shock.

A: ALLERGIES

- **Does the person have any known allergies?**

  Allergic reactions can lead to shock by causing abnormal relaxation of the blood vessels.

M: MEDICATIONS

- **Currently taking any medications?**

  Obtain a full medication list from the person or the family. Knowing the patient's medication list can help understand why the patient is in shock (such as heart medications). Overdose of blood pressure or seizure/convulsion medications can cause shock, and it may be more difficult to treat shock from any cause in patients taking these medications. Medications that thin the blood can worsen bleeding. Always ask about new medications in particular and recent dose changes to evaluate for allergic reaction or unexpected side effects.

P: PAST MEDICAL HISTORY

- **History of pregnancy or recent miscarriage or delivery?**

  Blood loss following delivery can be severe if the uterus does not contract well. Hidden blood loss leading to shock can occur with ruptured ectopic pregnancy, even in women who do not know they are pregnant. Any woman of childbearing age with shock should be evaluated for pregnancy.

- **History of recent surgery or induced abortion?**

  Internal bleeding or infection after surgery can lead to shock.

- **History of heart disease (heart attack or heart valve problems)?**

  Patients with heart disease are at risk for worsening heart function that may lead to shock or worsen shock from other causes.

- **Is there a history of HIV?**

  HIV increases the risk of infection.

L: LAST ORAL INTAKE

- **When did the person last eat or drink?**

  A person who is not eating or drinking well can develop severe dehydration, leading to shock.

E: EVENTS SURROUNDING ILLNESS

- **Has there been any recent trauma?**

  Trauma can cause hidden internal bleeding, tension pneumothorax, and bruising or bleeding around the heart, all of which may reduce blood flow and cause shock. In addition, trauma to the neck or back causing spinal cord injury can interfere with the blood vessels' ability to maintain blood pressure.

- **Has there been any recent illness?**

  Any infection can cause a blood infection that can spread throughout the body and lead to shock.

INTRO

ABCDE

TRAUMA

BREATHING

SHOCK

AMS

SKILLS

GLOSSARY

REFS & QUICK CARDS

Workbook question 1: Shock

Using the workbook section above, list six questions about signs and symptoms you would ask when taking a SAMPLE history.

1. _____

2. _____

3. _____

4. _____

5. _____

6. _____

CHECK: SECONDARY EXAMINATION FINDINGS IN SHOCK

A person with shock will have signs of poor perfusion, which may include a fast heart rate, a low systolic blood pressure, fast breathing, pale and cool skin, slow capillary refill, dizziness, confusion, altered mental status, decreased urine output or excessive sweating.

REMEMBER: Perfusion can be limited even before blood pressure falls, especially in the young. Low blood pressure with poor perfusion is a very serious sign.

Always assess ABCDE first. The initial ABCDE approach identifies and manages life-threatening conditions. The secondary exam looks for changes in the patient's condition or less obvious causes that may have been missed during ABCDE. If the secondary examination identifies an ABCDE condition, **STOP AND RETURN IMMEDIATELY TO ABCDE** to manage it.

REMEMBER: Children have different normal vital signs ranges, and children with shock may not have changes in vital signs until they are very ill. Always do a careful exam for any signs of shock.

- Check *breath sounds and respiratory rate:*
  - Abnormal or noisy breathing can indicate pneumonia as a source for system-wide infection causing shock.
  - High sugar levels can result in chemical imbalance (diabetic ketoacidosis) that the body tries to address by faster or deeper breathing. This condition may also result in sweet or 'fruity' smelling breath. Since elevated blood glucose levels cause increased urination, severe dehydration and shock can result.

- Check for *bleeding:*
  - All external bleeding should be controlled with direct pressure. [See SKILLS] Arterial bleeding may appear as pulsing or high pressure bleeding, and significant blood volume can be lost in minutes.

- Vaginal bleeding may be an important source of blood loss from pregnancy-related bleeding (even in those who think they are not pregnant) or from masses in the cervix or uterus.

▪ **Check *fluid status:***

In dehydration states, the patient may feel thirsty or may have dry lips and mouth, abnormal skin pinch, lethargy, and delayed capillary refill. Patients with heart failure can be in shock with fluid overload, and may have lower body swelling (usually in both legs), crackles on lung examination, and distended neck veins.

▪ **Check for *pale conjunctiva (the inside of the lower eyelid):***

No matter the person's skin color, the inside of the eyelid should appear pink and moist. If the inner portion of the eyelid (conjunctiva) is pale, it may indicate significant blood loss. You can compare the patient's conjunctiva to another healthy person or look at your own in a mirror.

▪ **Check *mental status:***

Confusion in a patient with other signs of poor perfusion suggests severe shock.

▪ **Check for *fever:***

Fever in a patient with shock suggests severe infection.

▪ **Check *blood sugar:***

Low blood glucose can sometimes look like shock. If you cannot check blood glucose, but the person has altered mental status, a history of diabetes or another reason to have low sugar (for example, is taking quinine for malaria, is very ill, or is very malnourished), give glucose. [See SKILLS]

▪ **Check for *severe abdominal pain or a very firm abdomen:***

If the person has severe abdominal pain, this can be a sign of bleeding or infection in the abdomen. In a patient who might be pregnant, this can be a sign of an ectopic pregnancy.

▪ **Check *urine:***

Check the urine colour and volume. Small amounts of darker urine may indicate substantial dehydration.

▪ **Check *stool:***

Any significant diarrhoea can cause dehydration. A large amount of watery, "rice-water" stool suggests cholera, which can rapidly cause severe dehydration and shock. Black, dark, or reddish colored stool can suggest stomach or intestinal bleeding.

- **Check for *malnourishment* [see SKILLS]:**

If the person appears malnourished, fluid must be adjusted [see SKILLS]. Be sure to ask about recent changes in weight.

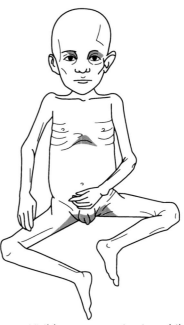

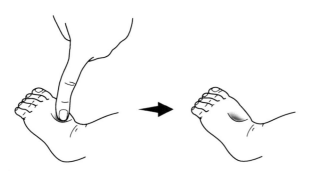

Assessing for pitting edema in children with malnutrition

Visible severe wasting in a child

- **Check for *swelling, rash or excessive sweating:***

Swelling of mouth or body can indicate an allergic reaction. Rashes can indicate allergic reaction (hives) or systemic infection. Swelling of both legs can indicate heart failure. Sweating may occur with moderate to severe shock.

Workbook question 2: Shock

Using the workbook section above, list what you need to check for in a person with shock.

1. _____

2. _____

3. _____

4. _____

5. _____

6. _____

7. _____

8. _____

9. _____

10. _____

INTRO

ABCDE

TRAUMA

BREATHING

SHOCK

AMS

SKILLS

GLOSSARY

REFS & QUICK CARDS

POSSIBLE CAUSES OF SHOCK

POOR PERFUSION DUE TO DILATED BLOOD VESSELS

CONDITION	SIGNS AND SYMPTOMS
Severe infection	• Fever • Tachycardia • Tachypnoea • May have hypotension • May or may not have obvious infectious source: visible skin infection, cough and crackles in one area of the lungs (often with tachypnoea), burning with urination, urine that is cloudy or foul smelling, or any focal pain in association with fever
Spinal cord injury	• History or signs of trauma • May have spinal pain/tenderness, vertebrae not in line, or crepitus (crunching) when you touch the spinal bones • Movement problems: paralysis, weakness, abnormal reflexes • Sensation problems: tingling ("pins and needles" sensation), loss of sensation • Unable to control urine and stools • Priapism • May have hypotension or bradycardia • Difficulty in breathing with an upper cervical spine injury
Severe allergic reaction	• Swelling of the mouth • Difficulty breathing with stridor and/or wheezing • Skin rash • Tachycardia • Hypotension

POOR PERFUSION DUE TO FLUID LOSS

CONDITION	SIGNS AND SYMPTOMS
Diabetic ketoacidosis (DKA)	• May have known history of diabetes • Rapid or deep breathing • Frequent urination • Sweet-smelling breath • High glucose in blood or urine • Dehydration
Severe dehydration	• Abnormal skin pinch • Decreased fluid consumption or increased fluid loss (vomiting, diarrhoea, excessive urination) • Dry mucous membranes • Tachycardia
Burn injury	• Red, white or black areas of skin depending on depth of burn • May have blistering • May have signs of inhalational injury

POOR PERFUSION DUE TO BLOOD LOSS	
CONDITION	**SIGNS AND SYMPTOMS**
External bleeding	• History of trauma • Visible bleeding • Use of blood-thinning medications
Large bone fracture	• History of trauma • Pain or abnormal movement of the pelvis, blood at opening of penis or rectum (pelvic fracture) • Deformity or crepitus of the femur, shortening of the leg with the injury (femur fracture)
Abdominal bleeding	• Bruising around the umbilicus or over the flanks can be a sign of internal bleeding • Abdominal pain • Very firm abdomen
Bleeding in the stomach or intestines	• Blood in vomit or stool • Black vomit or stool • History of alcohol use
Haemothorax	• Difficulty in breathing • Decreased breath sounds on affected side • Dull sounds with percussion on affected side • Shock (if large amount of blood)
Ectopic pregnancy	• History of pregnancy, missed menstrual cycle or any woman of childbearing age • Abdominal pain • Vaginal bleeding

Postpartum haemorrhage	• Recent delivery
	• Heavy vaginal bleeding:
	  – Pad or cloth soaked in <5 minutes
	  – Constant trickling blood
	  – Bleeding >250 ml
	  – Soft uterus/lower abdomen

POOR PERFUSION DUE TO PROBLEMS WITH THE HEART

CONDITION	SIGNS AND SYMPTOMS
Heart failure	• Difficulty breathing with exertion or when lying flat • Swelling to both legs • Distended neck veins • Crackles may be heard in the lungs • May have chest pain
Heart attack	• Pressure, tightness, pain or crushing feeling in the chest • Diaphoresis and mottled skin • Difficulty in breathing • Nausea or vomiting • Pain moving to jaw or arms • Signs of heart failure • History of smoking, heart disease, hypertension, diabetes, high cholesterol, family history of heart problems
Abnormal heart rhythm	• Very fast or very slow pulse • Irregular pulse
Heart valve problem	• History of rheumatic fever or heart disease • Murmur
Pericardial tamponade	• Signs of poor perfusion (tachycardia, tachypnoea, hypotension, pale skin, cold extremities, capillary refill greater than 3 seconds) • Distended neck veins • Muffled heart sounds • May have dizziness, confusion, altered mental status • History of tuberculosis, trauma, cancer, kidney failure

Tension pneumothorax	• Hypotension WITH the following:
	  – Difficulty breathing
	  – Absent breath sounds on affected side
	  – Hyperresonance with percussion on affected side
	  – Distended neck veins
	  – May have tracheal shift away from affected side

REMEMBER... hypoglycaemia can look like shock. Signs and symptoms include:

- Sweating (diaphoresis)
- Seizure/convulsion
- Blood glucose <3.5 mmol/L
- Altered mental status (ranging from confusion to unconsciousness)
- History of diabetes, malaria, or a severe illness, especially in children

Workbook Question 3: Shock

Using the workbook section above, list the possible cause of shock next to the history and physical findings below.

HISTORY AND PHYSICAL FINDINGS	LIKELY CAUSE
A 35-year-old woman presents with shock, fever and: • burning with urination • cloudy urine	
A 20-year-old woman presents with shock, abdominal pain and: • missed menstrual cycle • vaginal bleeding	
A 17-year-old man presents after a motor vehicle crash with shock, bruising to the pelvis and: • a femur fracture	

DO: MANAGEMENT

FIRST PERFORM ABCDE ASSESSMENT AND INTERVENE FOR LIFE-THREATENING CONDITIONS.

Start by giving IV fluid (normal saline or Ringer's Lactate in adults and children with normal nutritional status). Then work to address underlying causes. Place IV access rapidly (two large-bore IVs) and start IV fluids. Place IV access rapidly (two large-bore IVs), start IV fluids and assess response. Repeat with additional boluses if needed. [See SKILLS] If you cannot place an IV, immediately call for a provider who can place a nasogastric tube (a tube that goes from the nose into the stomach) or intraosseous line (a needle that is placed directly into the bone). See if the patient can safely take oral fluids in the meantime.

CAUTION! For severely malnourished or severely anaemic people, or anyone with signs of volume overload, do NOT follow the fluid protocol below. Use adjusted protocol. [See SKILLS]

INTRO

ABCDE

TRAUMA

BREATHING

SHOCK

AMS

SKILLS

GLOSSARY

REFS & QUICK CARDS

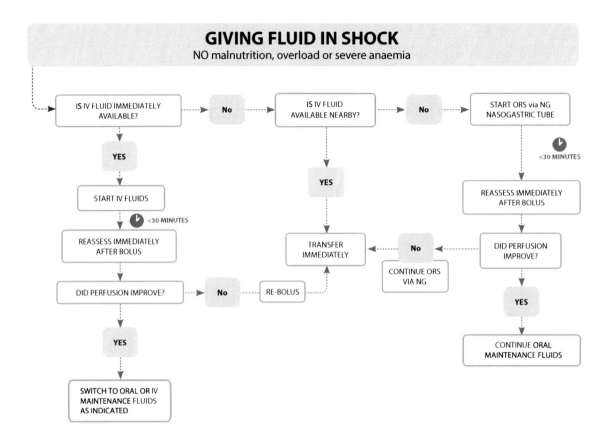

GIVING FLUID IN SHOCK
NO malnutrition, overload or severe anaemia

IS IV FLUID IMMEDIATELY AVAILABLE? → No → IS IV FLUID AVAILABLE NEARBY? → No → START ORS via NG NASOGASTRIC TUBE

YES → START IV FLUIDS → <30 MINUTES → REASSESS IMMEDIATELY AFTER BOLUS → DID PERFUSION IMPROVE? → No → RE-BOLUS

YES → SWITCH TO ORAL OR IV MAINTENANCE FLUIDS AS INDICATED

YES → TRANSFER IMMEDIATELY ← No ← CONTINUE ORS VIA NG ← DID PERFUSION IMPROVE?

<30 MINUTES → REASSESS IMMEDIATELY AFTER BOLUS → DID PERFUSION IMPROVE? → YES → CONTINUE ORAL MAINTENANCE FLUIDS

If vaginal bleeding after delivery (postpartum haemorrhage) is suspected as a cause of shock: ALL patients need rapid handover/transfer to an advanced obstetric provider. While arranging for transport and during transport, it is important to try to stop the bleeding. Give BOTH intramuscular and IV oxytocin. This is a loading dose. After these doses, continue oxytocin IV until one hour after the bleeding stops. [See SKILLS] Bleeding frequently happens if the uterus is not fully contracted (does not feel hard on palpation). Perform uterine massage [See SKILLS] until the uterus is hard. You should use BOTH oxytocin and uterine massage to stop the bleeding. If the placenta delivers, collect it in a leak-proof container and keep with the patient to allow the advanced obstetric provider to examine it. Visually check externally for a perineal or vaginal tear. If found, apply direct pressure with sterile gauze and put legs together. Even if the bleeding stops, these patients still need rapid handover/transfer to an advanced obstetric provider (see figure).

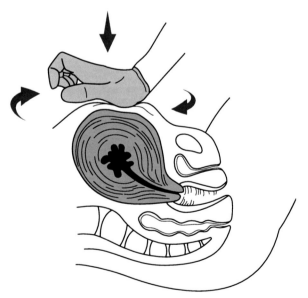

Uterine massage for postpartum hemorrhage

Postpartum Haemorrhage

1. Arrange immediate transfer to qualified obstetric provider!

2. Attempt to control bleeding while arranging and during transfer.

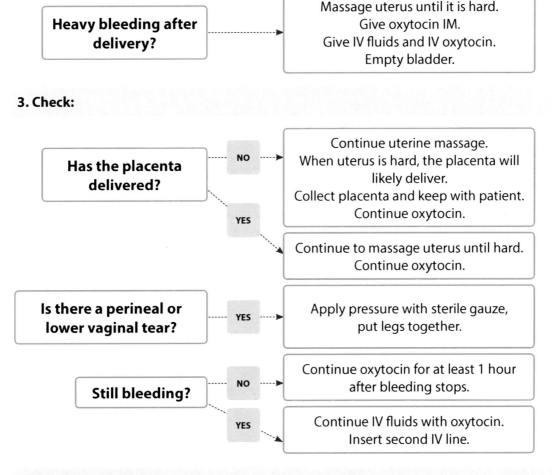

| Heavy bleeding after delivery? | ⇢ | Massage uterus until it is hard.
Give oxytocin IM.
Give IV fluids and IV oxytocin.
Empty bladder. |

3. Check:

| Has the placenta delivered? | NO → | Continue uterine massage.
When uterus is hard, the placenta will likely deliver.
Collect placenta and keep with patient.
Continue oxytocin. |
| | YES → | Continue to massage uterus until hard.
Continue oxytocin. |

| Is there a perineal or lower vaginal tear? | YES → | Apply pressure with sterile gauze, put legs together. |

| Still bleeding? | NO → | Continue oxytocin for at least 1 hour after bleeding stops. |
| | YES → | Continue IV fluids with oxytocin.
Insert second IV line. |

4. Transfer immediately

REMEMBER... fluid only addresses the immediate problem of perfusion. Patients with shock need rapid handover/transfer to a unit capable of addressing the causes of shock and providing advanced management, including transfusion.

REMEMBER... fluid status assessment is critical. Patients who have signs of poor perfusion but overall volume overload can be particularly difficult to manage. Patients with malnutrition, severe anaemia, and excess fluid in the lungs due to heart, liver, or kidney failure can present this way. These patients still need fluids, but the fluids must be given cautiously and, especially in malnourished children, according to a specific protocol. [See SKILLS]

INTRO

ABCDE

TRAUMA

BREATHING

SHOCK

AMS

SKILLS

GLOSSARY

REFS & QUICK CARDS

DO: MANAGEMENT OF SPECIFIC CONDITIONS

> - Always perform ABCDE first. Patients in shock need oxygen.
> - In all forms of shock, the primary management is administration of IV fluids appropriate for age and condition.
> - The specific conditions below require additional considerations.

CONDITION	MANAGEMENT CONSIDERATIONS
Burns	• Burns disrupt the skin barrier and can cause significant fluid losses that can lead to shock. These patients have different fluid replacement needs. [See SKILLS]
Hyperglycaemia	• If concern for diabetic ketoacidosis, treat with IV fluids. [See SKILLS] A person with diabetic ketoacidosis is extremely ill and requires rapid transfer to a unit where IV infusion and close monitoring are available.
Fever	• Give fluids and start antibiotics. [See SKILLS] If infectious diarrhoea (like cholera) is suspected, use gloves, aprons and relevant isolation precautions and report it to the local public health agency. If signs of poor perfusion do not improve with fluids, consider rapid handover/transfer.
Spinal cause	• Give IV fluids and refer for ongoing management at a unit that can provide spinal care. [See SKILLS]
Stomach or intestinal bleeding	• Start IV fluids and refer for blood transfusion. [See SKILLS]
Ectopic pregnancy	• Give IV fluids and refer for blood transfusion and obstetric care. [See SKILLS]
Postpartum haemorrhage	• Give oxytocin and IV fluids and plan for rapid transfer to facility with blood transfusion and obstetric care capabilities. • Give IV fluids and massage uterus until it is hard. [See SKILLS] • Give oxytocin. [See SKILLS] • If the placenta has delivered, collect it in a leak-proof container and keep with patient for inspection by advanced provider. • Check for perineal and vaginal tears and apply direct pressure.
Tension pneumothorax	• Perform needle decompression immediately to relieve the pressure, give oxygen and IV fluids. [See SKILLS] Any patient who has had a needle decompression will need rapid handover/transfer to a unit that can place a chest tube.
Pericardial tamponade	• Give IV fluids to help fill the heart against the building pressure in the heart sac. [See SKILLS] Plan for rapid handover/transfer to a provider who can drain the pericardial fluid.

CONDITION	MANAGEMENT CONSIDERATIONS
Suspected heart attack	• Give aspirin if indicated. Place an IV and give fluids, re-assessing the patient frequently. [See SKILLS] • While oxygen is no longer recommended in all patients with heart attack, it should initially be given in patients with shock or difficulty in breathing, even when heart attack is the suspected cause. • Plan for rapid handover/transfer to advanced provider.
Heart failure	• Give IV fluids more slowly, checking the lungs for crackles (fluid overload) frequently. Stop IV fluids if fluid overload develops (difficulty in breathing, crackles in the lungs, increased respiratory rate, increased heart rate). [See SKILLS] • Plan for rapid handover/transfer to an advanced provider.
Severe allergic reaction	• Give intramuscular adrenaline [See SKILLS]. These patients will also need IV access and fluids as their condition can rapidly worsen once the adrenaline wears off. You may give a second dose if the effects wear off. [See SKILLS] If the airway is swollen or there is difficulty in breathing, patients may need rapid transfer.
Traumatic injury or rapid blood loss suspected	• Stop the bleeding, give IV fluids, and conduct a thorough trauma assessment. [See SKILLS] Refer for blood transfusion and ongoing surgical management.

Workbook question 4: Shock

Using the workbook section above, list what you would do to manage this patient.

A 6-year-old boy is brought in with fever. He is in shock and does not appear malnourished. Your facility has supplies to put in an IV.

1. _____
2. _____
3. _____

A young man is brought in after a motorcycle crash. He has a large cut to his arm that is bleeding and there is a large pool of blood under him. He is in shock when you examine him.

1. _____
2. _____
3. _____

A 30-year-old woman is brought in after accidentally eating prawns. She has a known shellfish allergy, her body is covered in a red, itchy rash and she is in shock.

1. _____
2. _____
3. _____

INTRO

ABCDE

TRAUMA

BREATHING

SHOCK

AMS

SKILLS

GLOSSARY

REFS & QUICK CARDS

111

SPECIAL CONSIDERATIONS IN CHILDREN

Shock can occur quite rapidly in children and is life-threatening. Children have a relatively larger surface area (compared to their body volume) and are thus likely to become dehydrated more rapidly. Infants and young children are particularly at risk as they are unable to say when they are thirsty and cannot drink more on their own.

Assessing shock in children: The clinical definition of shock in children varies. The 2016 WHO guidelines for the care of critically ill children use the presence of three clinical features: cold extremities, capillary refill greater than 3 seconds, and weak and fast pulse. There are also other important signs of poor perfusion, including low blood pressure, fast breathing, altered mental status, and decreased urination (always ask parents how much urine the child is passing). [See SKILLS]

Signs of dehydration in children

- Very dry mouth and lips
- Lethargy (excessive drowsiness and slowness to respond), child not interactive
- Sunken eyes
- Small amounts of dark urine (ask about number of nappies for infants)
- Sunken fontanelles in infants under 1 year
- Delayed capillary refill (normal capillary refill is less than 3 seconds)
- Abnormal skin pinch [See SKILLS]
- Pallor (anaemia makes dehydration even more difficult to treat [See SKILLS])

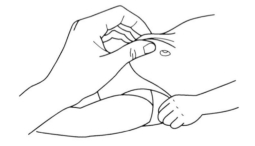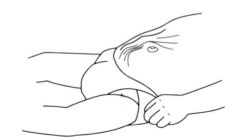

Abnormal skin pinch in a child

Common causes of shock and dehydration in children include:

- *Vomiting and diarrhoea:* Gastroenteritis causes sudden onset of vomiting and diarrhoea with some abdominal pain and fever. Large amount of watery diarrhoea may suggest cholera, and needs to be reported to public health authorities.

- *Vomiting without diarrhoea*: Vomiting without diarrhoea or fever may suggest raised pressure on the brain (trauma, tumour, brain swelling), or intestinal blockage. It is important to examine the child for signs of trauma. Vomiting associated with fever may suggest infection.

- *Overwhelming infection:* Fever can cause children to become dehydrated quickly. In addition, overwhelming infection can cause blood vessels to dilate, worsening shock.

Special management considerations:

- *Malnourishment:* Malnourished children are at high risk for hypoglycaemia and will need sugar in addition to fluids. Give specialized fluids if available. [See SKILLS] Give less IV fluid more slowly, and check the lungs for crackles (fluid overload) every 5 minutes. Stop IV fluids if fluid overload develops (crackles in the lungs, increased respiratory rate, increased heart rate). Switch to oral fluids as soon as signs of poor perfusion improve. These patients need rapid handover/transfer over to an advanced provider at a centre with blood transfusion capabilities.

Workbook question 5: Shock

Using the workbook section above, list signs of severe dehydration in children.

1. _____

2. _____

3. _____

4. _____

5. _____

6. _____

7. _____

8. _____

DISPOSITION CONSIDERATIONS

- People with shock can worsen and die quickly. They must be monitored very closely.

- Additionally, the same illnesses that cause shock interfere with the body's ability to manage fluids, so these patients must be monitored very closely for signs of difficulty in breathing.

- Patients with shock may be confused and anxious. Ensure they are safe and contained during transfer.

- Patients with shock are often transferred for transfusion or general or obstetric surgery. Always communicate directly with the receiving facility to make sure that these resources are actually available at the time of transfer.

INTRO
ABCDE
TRAUMA
BREATHING
SHOCK
AMS
SKILLS
GLOSSARY
REFS & QUICK CARDS

FACILITATOR-LED CASE SCENARIOS

These case scenarios will be presented in small groups. One participant will be identified as the lead and will be assessed while the rest of the group writes the responses in the workbook. To complete a case scenario, participants must identify the critical findings and management needed, and formulate a one-line summary for handover, including assessment findings and interventions. You should use the Quick Card for these scenarios while being assessed.

CASE #1: ADULT SHOCK

A 48-year-old male with a history of alcohol abuse is brought in by his wife to be evaluated for weakness. His wife states that he has been having very dark stools for the past 2 days and now cannot stand up.

1. What do you need to do in your initial approach?

2. Use the ABCDE approach to assess and manage this patient. Ask the facilitator about look, listen and feel findings; use the Quick Card for reference as needed.

	ASSESSMENT	FINDINGS	INTERVENTION NEEDED?		INTERVENTIONS TO PERFORM:
AIRWAY			YES	NO	
BREATHING			YES	NO	
CIRCULATION			YES	NO	
DISABILITY			YES	NO	
EXPOSURE			YES	NO	

3. Formulate one sentence to summarize this patient for handover.

CASE #2: PAEDIATRIC SHOCK

The patient is a 4-year-old girl brought in by her mother. She has been having almost constant diarrhoea for the past 3 days and vomiting every time she tries to drink anything. The mother thinks she may have had a fever as well. She has no signs of malnutrition.

1. What do you need to do in your initial approach?

2. Use the ABCDE approach to assess and manage this patient. Ask the facilitator about look, listen and feel findings; use the Quick Card for reference as needed.

	ASSESSMENT	FINDINGS	INTERVENTION NEEDED?		INTERVENTIONS TO PERFORM:
AIRWAY			YES	NO	
BREATHING			YES	NO	
CIRCULATION			YES	NO	
DISABILITY			YES	NO	
EXPOSURE			YES	NO	

3. Formulate one sentence to summarize this patient for handover.

INTRO
ABCDE
TRAUMA
BREATHING
SHOCK
AMS
SKILLS
GLOSSARY
REFS & QUICK CARDS

MULTIPLE CHOICE QUESTIONS

Answer the questions below. Questions and answers will be discussed in the session.

1. A 7-year-old boy has had lethargy, vomiting and diarrhoea for the past 4 days. His vital signs are: blood pressure 80/40 mmHg, heart rate 140 beats per minute, respiratory rate 18 breaths per minute. The patient vomits when you try to give anything by mouth. What is your most immediate management?

   A.   Start an IV line and give fluids

   B.   Continue to attempt oral rehydration

   C.   Place a nasogastric (NG) tube and hydrate through it

   D.   Rapidly transfer to a referral hospital

2. You are taking care of a 28-year-old man who was shot in the abdomen. He is lethargic and the vital signs are as follows: blood pressure 80/40 mmHg, heart rate 130 beats per minute, respiratory rate 20 breaths per minute. There is heavy bleeding from the gunshot wound and the abdomen is rigid and tender. What is the first intervention you should give this patient?

   A.   IV fluids

   B.   Intraosseous line

   C.   Surgery

   D.   Adrenaline

3. A child that presents with sunken eyes, small amounts of dark urine, dry mucous membranes and abnormal skin pinch testing is most likely suffering from:

   A.   Pneumonia

   B.   Head injury

   C.   Dehydration

   D.   Hypoglycaemia

4. A 60-year-old man states he has been weak and dizzy for the past week. His vital signs are: blood pressure 90/50 mmHg, heart rate 125 beats per minute, respiratory rate 16 breaths per minute. His skin is cool and pale. He states that his stools have been black for the past 2 days. What is the most likely cause of his shock?

   A.   Stomach bleeding

   B.   Abdominal trauma

   C.   Dehydration

   D.   Severe infection

5. You are assessing a 23-year-old man who was stabbed in the chest. You expose the chest to find one stab wound in the right chest with minor bleeding. He is complaining of severe difficulty in breathing and there are no lung sounds on the right side. His neck veins are distended and his skin is cool and sweaty. His vital signs are: blood pressure 86/56 mmHg, heart rate 136 beats per minute, respiratory rate 28 breaths per minute. What is your next step?

A. Chest tube placement

B. Needle decompression

C. Blood transfusion

D. Start IV fluids

INTRO

ABCDE

TRAUMA

BREATHING

SHOCK

AMS

SKILLS

GLOSSARY

REFS & QUICK CARDS

Notes

Module 5:
Approach to altered mental status

Objectives

On completing this module you should be able to:

1. recognize key history findings suggestive of different causes of altered mental status;

2. recognize key physical findings suggestive of different causes of altered mental status;

3. list high-risk causes of altered mental status in adults and children;

4. perform critical actions for high-risk causes of altered mental status.

Essential skills

- Glasgow Coma Scale
- AVPU assessment
- Recovery position
- Oxygen administration
- IV cannula insertion
- IV fluid resuscitation
- Snake-bite management
- Spinal immobilization

KEY TERMS

Write the definition using the Glossary at the back of the workbook.

Altered mental status:

_____

Coma:

_____

Confusion:

_____

Convulsion:

_____

Cyanosis:

_____

INTRO

ABCDE

TRAUMA

BREATHING

SHOCK

AMS

SKILLS

GLOSSARY

REFS & QUICK CARDS

Delirium:

Dementia:

Diabetic ketoacidosis (DKA):

Eclampsia:

Envenomation:

Human Immunodeficiency Virus (HIV):

Hypoglycaemia:

Hypoxia:

Ingestion:

Kangaroo care:

Large-bore IV:

Level of consciousness:

Orientation:

Psychosis:

 Rabies:

Seizure:

Stroke:

Overview

Altered mental status (AMS) is a term used for a range of presentations, from sudden or gradual changes in behaviour to disorientation, confusion and coma. Changes in mental status and/or level of consciousness may be due to conditions that affect the brain (such as lack of oxygen or glucose; or shock causing lack of perfusion) or problems with the brain itself (such as infection, inflammation or injury). While chronic psychiatric problems and dementia can cause changes in mental status, altered mental status is often an indication of severe disease, and other life-threatening causes must always be considered. The presence of delirium – a rapidly changing state of confusion with agitation, loss of focus and inability to interact appropriately – always requires a full assessment. Always ask family/friends about baseline mental status when possible.

The goal of INITIAL ASSESSMENT is to identify rapidly reversible causes of altered mental status, and to recognize dangerous conditions requiring transfer.

The goal of ACUTE MANAGEMENT is to ensure that blood, oxygen and glucose reach the brain; and to protect the brain from additional injury.

This module will guide you through:

- ABCDE key elements
- ASK: key history findings (SAMPLE history)
- CHECK: secondary exam findings
- Possible causes
- DO: Management
- Special considerations in children
- Disposition considerations

REMEMBER...

- ALWAYS **START WITH THE ABCDE APPROACH**, intervening as needed.
- **Then do a SAMPLE history.**
- **Then do a secondary exam.**

INTRO

ABCDE

TRAUMA

BREATHING

SHOCK

AMS

SKILLS

GLOSSARY

REFS & QUICK CARDS

ABCDE: KEY ELEMENTS FOR ALTERED MENTAL STATUS

For the person with altered mental status, the following are key elements that should be considered in the ABCDE approach.

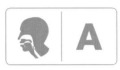

AIRWAY
People with altered mental status may not be able to protect their airways and may be at risk of choking on vomit.

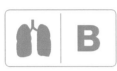

BREATHING
Hypoxia (lack of oxygen) can be a cause of altered mental status. Search for any signs of difficulty breathing, or cyanosis (blue colouring of the skin). Abnormal breathing can reflect **diabetic ketoacidosis** or **poisoning**.

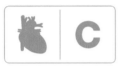

CIRCULATION
Lack of perfusion to the brain can cause altered mental status. Look for and manage signs of **shock** (low blood pressure, elevated heart rate, delayed capillary refill).

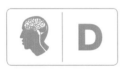

DISABILITY
Check AVPU or GCS (in trauma). Look for abnormal glucose (**hypoglycaemia or hyperglycaemia** can cause altered mental status). Very small pupils suggest **opioid overdose or poisoning** (consider pesticides). Very dilated pupils suggest **stimulant drug** use. Unequal pupils suggest an **increased pressure on the brain**. If the patient can follow commands, test for strength and sensation in face, arms and legs. Weakness or loss of sensation on one side suggests a **mass, bleeding, or blocked blood vessels in the brain (stroke)**, though **hypoglycemia** can also present this way. Altered mental status with general muscle weakness may suggest **salt (electrolyte) imbalance** in the blood. Look for abnormal repetitive movements or shaking on one or both sides of the body (**seizure/ convulsion**) – this may be due to a tumour, bleeding, brain infection, hypoglycaemia, or salt (electrolyte) imbalance.

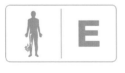

EXPOSURE
Remember that patients with altered mental status may not report their history accurately. Examine the entire body for **infections, rashes**, and any evidence of **trauma, bites** or **stings**. Needle marks on the arms may suggest **drugs** as a cause.

ASK: KEY HISTORY FINDINGS FOR PATIENTS WITH ALTERED MENTAL STATUS

Use the SAMPLE approach to obtain a history from the patient and/or family. It is important to obtain a history from bystanders, friends or family as it may be difficult to obtain accurate history from a confused patient. For example, a person with hypoglycaemia may be too confused to relate a history of diabetes.

If the history identifies an ABCDE condition, STOP AND RETURN IMMEDIATELY TO ABCDE to manage it.

S: SIGNS AND SYMPTOMS

- **How does the current condition compare to baseline mental status?**

  Always ask family/friends about baseline mental status when possible.

- **Is there difficulty breathing?**

  Altered mental status associated with difficulty in breathing may indicate lack of oxygen to the brain.

- **Is there headache?**

  Headache with altered mental status can indicate infection, tumour or bleeding.

- **Is there vomiting/diarrhoea?**

  Vomiting without diarrhoea can be a sign of increased pressure in the brain. Any source of dehydration, including vomiting and diarrhoea, may cause altered mental status from poor perfusion. Vomiting and diarrhoea can also cause hypoglycaemia leading to altered mental status.

- **Has there been any dizziness or fainting?**

  These may be signs of poor perfusion (lack of oxygenated blood) to the brain.

- **When did the symptoms start? Do they come and go? How long do they last? Have they changed over time?**

  Rapid onset of altered mental status may suggest infection, inflamation, bleeding or drugs/toxic exposures. A more gradual onset (over weeks or months) may indicate a space-occupying lesion in the brain, such as a tumour or slow bleeding in the brain. Altered mental status that comes and goes with normal intervals between episodes may suggest other causes, such as seizures/convulsions or psychiatric disease.

- **Has there been any recent fever?**

  Any person with altered mental status and fever may have an infection. Brain infections often present with altered mental status and fever. In small children and the elderly, any serious infection, such as urine, lung, or blood infection can cause altered mental status. Also consider prolonged outdoor exposure, poisonings, medications and drugs as these may present with fever as well. Very high fever itself from any source may cause altered mental status.

- **Is there any weakness, clumsiness or difficulty walking?**

  Change in mental status with weakness or sensory loss in one area of the body, or problems with walking and balance, suggest that the altered mental status comes from a cause in the brain itself, such as a stroke or tumour.

- **Is there neck pain or stiffness?**

  Fluid that circulates around the brain also circulates around the spinal cord, meaning any bleeding, inflammation or infection in the brain (meningitis, encephalitis) can also cause neck pain and stiffness.

INTRO
ABCDE
TRAUMA
BREATHING
SHOCK
AMS
SKILLS
GLOSSARY
REFS & QUICK CARDS

- **Is there a recent history of trauma or falls?**

  Bleeding in or around the brain can cause altered mental status some days after an injury. Remember that chronic alcohol drinkers and the elderly are more prone to brain bleeding and may not remember falls. Always consider slow bleeding around the brain as a cause, even several days after a fall, and consider unwitnessed trauma in a patient who is found altered with no known cause.

- **Has there been any recent depression or changes in behaviour?**

  Drug and alcohol use or psychiatric problems can present as altered mental status. Always consider the possibility of a suicide attempt by poisoning.

- **Does anyone else from the same family or location have symptoms?**

  Gaseous poisoning, like carbon monoxide poisoning, can cause altered mental status in multiple people. Carbon monoxide poisoning is usually seen in cold climates when people use indoor heating.

A: ALLERGIES

- **Any allergies or recent exposure to a known allergen?**

  Severe allergic reactions (anaphylaxis) may present with altered mental status due to low blood oxygen levels or poor blood circulation to the brain as a result of shock.

M: MEDICATIONS

- **Currently taking any medications?**

  Many common medications can cause altered mental status as a side effect, including those for seizures/convulsions, pain and sleeping. Ask about new medications and changed doses, and consider medication interactions. A medication list should be collected and can provide clues for underlying disease (such as convulsions, liver disease, diabetes) if the person cannot communicate. Opioid medications (such as morphine, pethidine and heroin) can cause altered mental status.

P: PAST MEDICAL HISTORY

- **History of diabetes?**

  In any patient with diabetes and altered mental status, suspect diabetic crisis, or low blood sugar caused by medications. Recent increase in urine output, increased thirst, and fast or deep breathing suggest diabetic crisis (diabetic ketoacidosis).

- **History of heart disease?**

  Heart attack can cause decreased blood flow and oxygen to the brain leading to confusion. Those with heart disease are also at an increased risk of stroke.

- **History of stroke?**

  Altered mental status in a patient with a history of stroke may suggest an additional stroke or bleeding in the brain. Be sure to ask people who know the patient about his or her usual mental and neurological status. Symptoms of old stroke may return with severe illness of any kind.

- **History of high blood pressure?**

  High blood pressure increases the risk for bleeding in and around the brain (such as stroke).

- **History of seizure/convulsion?**

  Altered mental status in a patient with a history of seizures/convulsions may suggest that the patient is having or recovering from a convulsion. If there is a history of epilepsy (primary seizure/convulsion disorder), ask about regular medication and any recent dose changes or missed doses. With a witnessed convulsion, ask about fall or head trauma. Always ask if the convulsion was the same or different compared to prior. Remember that recovery of normal mental status after convulsions usually takes only a half hour to several hours at most, though patients may feel tired for longer. Longer altered mental status suggests another cause.

- **History of HIV infection?**

  Altered mental status in a person with HIV may suggest infection in or around the brain (meningitis, encephalitis).

- **History of tuberculosis?**

  Tuberculosis can infect the brain and cause altered mental status.

- **History of liver or kidney failure?**

  Liver or kidney failure can cause problems with the clearing of toxins and waste from the blood, which can lead to altered mental status.

- **History of heavy alcohol use?**

  Alcohol intoxication and alcohol withdrawal can present with altered mental status. People with a history of heavy alcohol use also have a high risk for head injury (and may not remember falls) and hypoglycaemia, both of which can cause altered mental status.

- **Use of drugs of abuse?**

  Several drugs of abuse cause altered mental status, including stimulants, sedatives and opioids.

- **History of pregnancy?**

  High blood pressure during pregnancy can lead to eclampsia (or seizures/convulsions and high blood pressure) during pregnancy.

L: LAST ORAL INTAKE

- **When did the person last eat or drink?**

  Low blood glucose levels and dehydration can cause altered mental status.

INTRO

ABCDE

TRAUMA

BREATHING

SHOCK

AMS

SKILLS

GLOSSARY

REFS & QUICK CARDS

E: EVENTS SURROUNDING ILLNESS

- **Recent trauma?**

  Both head injury and poor perfusion resulting from blood loss can cause altered mental status.

- **Recent travel to areas where certain types of infections might be more common?**

  Specific infections that can cause altered mental status may be more common in certain areas. Malaria is a key consideration in many areas.

- **Recent exposures: contact with a sick person, recent bites, chemical exposures, hot or cold environments etc.?**

  Sick contacts may suggest infectious cause. Chemical exposures (such as pesticides) or bites may suggest intoxication or envenomation. Altered mental status can be caused by both very low and very high body temperatures.

- **Recent alcohol or drug use?**

  Both alcohol intoxication and alcohol withdrawal can cause altered mental status. Methamphetamines and cocaine may cause severe agitation, while heroin (and other opioids) may cause lethargy and coma. See also "Past medical history" section above.

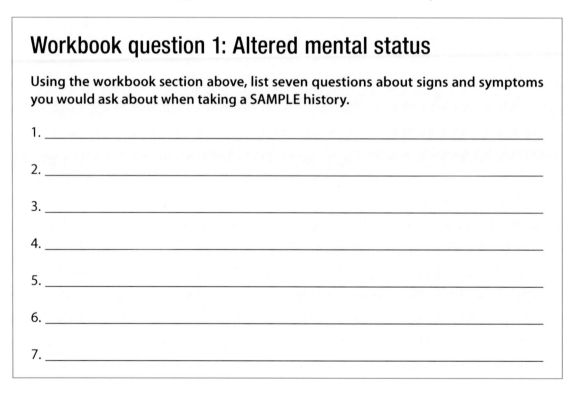

Workbook question 1: Altered mental status

Using the workbook section above, list seven questions about signs and symptoms you would ask about when taking a SAMPLE history.

1. _____

2. _____

3. _____

4. _____

5. _____

6. _____

7. _____

CHECK: SECONDARY EXAMINATION FINDINGS IN ALTERED MENTAL STATUS

A person with altered mental status may be unable to answer questions, and clues to the cause may only be found during the physical examination. Always assess ABCDE first. The initial ABCDE approach identifies and manages life-threatening conditions. The secondary examination looks for changes in the patient's condition or less obvious causes that may have been missed during ABCDE. If the secondary examination identifies an ABCDE condition, **STOP AND RETURN IMMEDIATELY TO ABCDE** to manage it.

- **Check for *safety:***

  Agitated and violent behaviour is a common presentation. It is very important to identify and treat the underlying cause if possible, while prioritizing the safety of the patient and providers. Keep calm and work as a team. Ensure that the space is safe from possible weapons and make sure that the patient is not between you and the door. Avoid making the patient feel threatened. Do not sit too close and speak with a calm, soft and sympathetic voice. Continually explain what is happening. Many aggressive patients will cooperate when faced with a team, so call for help and approach a patient as a group if necessary. Check vital signs, including temperature and glucose, and treat abnormalities. Call for help early and arrange handover/transfer to an advanced provider.

- **Check and monitor *level of consciousness* with the AVPU scale:**
  - **A: A**lert
  - **V:** Responds to **V**oice
  - **P:** Responds to **P**ain
  - **U: U**nresponsive

  AVPU tests the person's ability to respond to stimuli. A person who is not intoxicated and who has no illness or injury affecting the brain will usually be alert without being prompted. Patients who only respond when prompted by voice or pain require further assessment of the neurological system. [See SKILLS]

- **In trauma, check *Glasgow Coma Scale:***

  Check and monitor the Glasgow Coma Scale. [See SKILLS]

- **Check the *blood glucose level:***

  Hypoglycaemia can cause altered mental status. Diabetic ketoacidosis can present with hyperglycaemia and altered mental status.

- **Check the *pupils:***

  Very small pupils and slow breathing suggests opioid overdose. Very large (dilated) pupils suggest stimulant drug use. Unequal pupils suggest increased pressure on the brain.

- **Check for *orientation:***

  If the patient is alert and responds to voice, ask simple questions (for example: What is your name? Where are you? What time is it? What day of the week is it?).

- **Check for *trauma:***

  Any patient with altered mental status and history or evidence of trauma should be considered to have a possible head injury – even if the trauma occurred several days before. Bruising around the eyes, behind the ears, or leaking of clear fluid from the nose or ears suggests head injury with skull fracture.

- **Check *temperature:***

  Fever should raise concerns about an infectious cause, and fever with stiff neck suggests an infection in or around the brain. Poisonings, medication overdoses, alcohol withdrawal

INTRO

ABCDE

TRAUMA

BREATHING

SHOCK

AMS

SKILLS

GLOSSARY

REFS & QUICK CARDS

and changes in body hormones can also present with fever. Hypothermia may indicate infection, low body hormone levels (e.g., thyroid) or exposure to wet or cold environments.

- **Check for *stiff neck (Remember, if you suspect trauma, do not move the neck):***

  Stiff neck is suggestive of infection (meningitis) or bleeding around the brain. If you suspect infection, anyone who comes in contact with the patient should wear a mask.

- **Check *strength and sensation:***

  If the patient can follow commands, test for strength and sensation in face, arms and legs. Weakness or loss of sensation on one side suggests a mass, bleeding or blocked blood vessels in the brain (stroke), though hypoglycaemia can also present this way. Altered mental status with general muscle weakness may suggest salt (electrolyte) imbalance in the blood.

- **Check for *signs of dehydration:***

  Dehydration can cause altered mental status. Check for dry mouth and abnormal skin pinch. Dehydration may also suggest diabetic ketoacidosis.

- **Check the *abdomen:***

  Feel if the liver is enlarged or tender. A palpable or tender liver suggests liver disease.

- **Check the *skin:***

  Cool, pale, and moist skin suggests shock or hypoglycaemia. Yellow skin (jaundice) suggests liver disease. Bruising suggests trauma. Rashes can indicate systemic infection. Check for bites and stings.

- **Monitor for *changes in mental status:***

  People who are initially confused and rapidly return to normal without treatment may have had a seizure/convulsion or head trauma. People with altered mental status require close monitoring to make sure they do not worsen again. (This can happen in patients who have low blood sugar or head trauma).

Workbook question 2: Altered mental status

Using the workbook section above, list five secondary examination findings you would check for in a patient with altered mental status.

1. _____

2. _____

3. _____

4. _____

5. _____

POSSIBLE CAUSES OF ALTERED MENTAL STATUS

RAPIDLY REVERSIBLE CAUSES	
CONDITION	**SIGNS AND SYMPTOMS**
Hypoglycaemia	• Sweating (diaphoresis) • Seizures/convulsions • Blood glucose <3.5 mmol/L • History of diabetes, malaria, or severe illness, especially in children • Mental status improves quickly with glucose
Severe dehydration	• Signs of poor perfusion • Abnormal skin pinch • Decreased ability to drink fluids, or fluid loss • Dry mucous membranes
Heat stroke	• Prolonged exposure to heat and sun • High body temperature, very warm skin • May or may not be sweating (diaphoretic)
Hypoxia	• Shortness of breath • Low blood oxygen levels • Cyanosis

INFECTION	
CONDITION	**SIGNS AND SYMPTOMS**
Cerebral malaria	• Fever • Rapid malaria test or smear positive • In or from an area with malaria
Inflammation/infection around the brain (meningitis, encephalitis, brain abscess, bleeding)	• Fever • Neck stiffness • Rash • Eye pain with looking at light/sensitivity to light • Headache • Known infectious epidemic or exposure • History of HIV or TB infection
Severe infection	• Fever • Tachycardia • Tachypnoea • May have hypotension • Signs of infection: visible infection in the skin, cough and crackles in one area of the lungs (often with tachypnoea), burning with urination or urine that is cloudy (not clear), or any focal pain in association with fever
CONDITION	**SIGNS AND SYMPTOMS**
Rabies	• Agitation • Fear of drinking (hydrophobia) • Drooling • Weakness • History of animal bite

METABOLIC	
CONDITION	**SIGNS AND SYMPTOMS**
Diabetic ketoacidosis (DKA)	• History of diabetes • Rapid or deep breathing • Frequent urination • Sweet smelling breath • High glucose in blood or urine • Dehydration

TOXIC	
CONDITION	**SIGNS AND SYMPTOMS**

Alcohol or drug intoxication or withdrawal	• Known alcohol or drug use
	• Injection marks, drugs found on patients
	• Alcohol – breath smells of alcohol, reddened face
	  – Acutely intoxicated (drunk)
	  – Withdrawal (convulsions, confusion, tachycardia)
	  – Chronic use (balance problems, confusion)
	• Opioids:
	  – Acutely intoxicated (lethargy, very small pupils and slow breathing)
	  – Withdrawal (agitation, sweating, diarrhoea, vomiting)
	• Other drugs may cause large pupils, agitation, sweating, fever

Pesticide poisoning	• History of exposure • Very small pupils • Diarrhoea • Vomiting • Diaphoresis
Snake bite	• Snake bite history • Bite marks in a setting with venomous snakes • Oedema • Blistering of the skin • Bruising • Hypotension • Paralysis • Seizures • Bleeding from wounds
Medication reaction or dosing issue	• New medications or recent change in dose
Gaseous poisoning	• History consistent with possible exposure • Multiple people with symptoms • Headache

OTHER CAUSES	
CONDITION	**SIGNS AND SYMPTOMS**
Seizures/convulsions	• Known history of seizures/convulsions • Bitten tongue • Urinated on self • Gradual improvement over minutes or hours • If pregnant, consider eclampsia
Increased pressure on the brain (trauma, tumour, bleeding or brain swelling)	• Headache • Seizures/convulsions • Nausea, vomiting • Unequal pupils • Weakness on one side of the body or speech problems
Liver disease	• History of alcohol abuse or liver disease • Enlarged abdomen with thin arms, yellow coloring to the skin and eyes (jaundice), or hypoglycaemia
Kidney disease	• High blood pressure • Oedema or swelling in the legs • Decreased or no urine if severe
Head trauma	• Visual changes, loss of memory, vomiting, headache • History of recent trauma • Scalp lacerations and/or skull deformity • Bruising to head (particularly around eyes or behind ears) • Blood or clear fluid coming from nose or ears • Unequal pupils or weakness on one side of the body • Seizures/convulsions

ADDITIONAL CONSIDERATIONS IN CHILDREN	
CONDITION	**SIGNS AND SYMPTOMS**
Ingestions of chemicals or toxins	• Common in younger children • History of medications or substances found around child

INTRO

ABCDE

TRAUMA

BREATHING

SHOCK

AMS

SKILLS

GLOSSARY

REFS & QUICK CARDS

Workbook question 3: Altered mental status

Using the workbook section above, list the possible cause of altered mental status from the history and physical findings below.

HISTORY AND PHYSICAL FINDINGS	LIKELY CAUSE
A 15-year-old girl presents with altered mental status, fever and: • neck stiffness • eye pain when looking at light • headache	
A 45-year-old man presents with altered mental status, and deep, rapid breathing and: • frequent urination • sweet-smelling breath • high glucose in blood or urine • dehydration	

DO: MANAGEMENT

FIRST PERFORM ABCDE ASSESSMENT AND INTERVENE FOR LIFE-THREATENING CONDITIONS.

NOTE: If the airway is clear, and there is no evidence of trauma, place the patient in the recovery position to avoid getting fluid or vomit in the lungs. [See SKILLS]

CONDITION	MANAGEMENT CONSIDERATIONS
Hypoxia	Give oxygen. Look for underlying cause. [See SKILLS]
Hypoglycaemia	Treat with glucose. [See SKILLS]
Hyperglycaemia	If concern for diabetic ketoacidosis, treat with IV fluids. [See SKILLS] A person with diabetic ketoacidosis is extremely ill and requires rapid transfer to a unit where IV infusion and close monitoring are available.
Fever (hyperthermia) with altered mental status	Start antibiotics. Severe infections may require treatment by an advanced provider. Include malaria testing and treatment in endemic areas. Also consider poisoning and envenomation. Treat high fever with paracetamol. [See SKILLS] For severe temperature elevation, spray with cool water mist, fan and give IV fluids. Avoid shivering.
Hypothermia	Move to warm environment, remove wet clothing, warm with blankets and warm IV fluid.

CONDITION	MANAGEMENT CONSIDERATIONS
Bleeding or other cause of increased pressure on the brain	If no trauma, raise the head of the bed to 30 degrees. If trauma is suspected ensure spinal immobilization. [See SKILLS]
Opioid overdose	Administer naloxone. [See SKILLS] Naloxone effects last approximately 1 hour. Most opioids last longer and patients may need repeat naloxone dosing. Consider this when planning ongoing care and re-assess the person frequently.
Active seizure/convulsion	Treat with benzodiazepine and monitor the person closely to check for slow breathing. Check glucose or give glucose if you are unable to check. Place patient in recovery position if no trauma suspected. [See SKILLS] If the patient continues to seize or does not wake up between seizures, arrange for rapid transfer to an advanced provider and monitor the airway.
Pregnant with active seizure/convulsion	This could be eclampsia. Arrange rapid handover/transfer to a specialist unit and give magnesium sulphate. Monitor the patient closely for signs of toxicity. [See SKILLS] If any of these occur, do not give additional doses of magnesium.
Alcohol withdrawal	Always check glucose and give as needed. Treat withdrawal with a benzodiazepine. [See SKILLS] Monitor the airway closely.
Poisoning or envenomation	Try to identify the poison and refer to an advanced provider for specific treatments. If pesticide poisoning, make sure the patient has been decontaminated, and monitor the airway closely as the secretions can cause obstruction. Snake bites should be treated as described in the "Wound Management" section [see SKILLS] and referred as soon as possible for antivenom.
Rabies	There is no specific treatment for rabies. Symptomatic rabies is almost always fatal. See TRAUMA for management of suspected exposure from animal bite.
Violent or very agitated patient	Protect the patient from harming self or others. Ensure that staff have a clear exit path (do not place the patient between staff and the door). Remove potential weapons and unsafe objects. Call for help from colleagues, family members, and security if needed. Speak in a calm, soft, non-threatening tone. Explain what is happening at each stage of care. Do not confront or judge. Consider other causes: check glucose and vital signs including temperature and oxygen saturation. Treat abnormalities. Arrange for safe handover/transport to advanced provider.
Trauma	Assess GCS, immobilize the spine and evaluate for signs of increased pressure on the brain. [See SKILLS]

INTRO

ABCDE

TRAUMA

BREATHING

SHOCK

AMS

SKILLS

GLOSSARY

REFS & QUICK CARDS

SPECIAL CONSIDERATIONS

MANAGEMENT OF ACTIVE CONVULSIONS

- Check ABCDE.
- Maintain the airway – do not put anything in the mouth.
- Give oxygen if concern for hypoxia or prolonged seizure/convulsion.
- Place patient on his/her side, if possible.
- Protect the patient from harm or further injury.
- Check glucose or give glucose (if unable to check).
- Give a benzodiazepine.
- If pregnant and seizing, give magnesium sulphate.
- If no response, give another dose of benzodiazepine (repeat three times if needed) and monitor for low blood pressure and slow breathing.
- If the patient does not wake between seizure/convulsions, consider this a life-threatening condition. Arrange for rapid handover/transfer to an advanced provider.
- If the seizures/convulsions stop, place patient in recovery position and monitor closely.

Workbook question 4: Altered mental status

Using the workbook section above, list what you would do to manage these patients.

CONDITION	MANAGEMENT
A 3-year-old child presents with altered mental status and a blood glucose of 2 mmol/L.	1. _____
A 25-year-old woman is brought in with jerky movements and you suspect an active seizure/convulsion.	1. _____ 2. _____ 3. _____
A 50-year-old man is brought in following a fall from a roof. He has a headache and altered mental status.	1. _____ 2. _____

SPECIAL CONSIDERATIONS IN CHILDREN

Children with altered mental status may have seemingly mild signs such as sleeping more than usual or being less interactive. Manage ABCDE first, and then look for and manage causes of altered mental status. Remember that very ill or injured children may have normal vital signs until they rapidly deteriorate.

Hypoglycaemia occurs frequently in severely ill children and is a common cause of altered mental status in children. Check blood glucose (or give glucose if you are unable to check) in any child with altered mental status.

Hypoxia can occur as a result of many conditions, including respiratory infections and shock; birth hypoxia is a consideration in newborns.

Hyperthermia with altered mental status suggests infection, but can also be seen with excessive heat exposure, exercise, seizure/convulsion, hormonal imbalance and some medications and poisons.

Hypothermia with altered mental status can also suggest infection, particularly in infants, but can be due to drug intoxication, exposure to cold or hormonal imbalance. Young infants are more affected by variation in temperature. Keep the child warm by using blankets and a hat to prevent heat loss and using skin-to-skin contact (also called "kangaroo care") with a family member 24-hours per day while ill.

Seizures/convulsions can be due to fever alone but (as in adults) can also suggest infection, hypoglycaemia or hyponatremia (low sodium). Do not delay antibiotics in patients with suspected serious bacterial infection. Always consider trauma.

Infection in or around the brain can cause altered mental status. Look for a bulging or swollen fontanelle (in a child under 1 year) and/or rash to the legs and lower abdomen, which can indicate infection or increased pressure on the brain. Do not delay antibiotics in children with suspected serious bacterial infection.

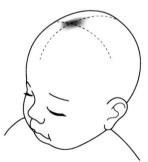

Flat fontanelle   *Bulging fontanelle*

Poor perfusion can cause altered mental status. Children can become dehydrated very quickly. Check for signs of dehydration: abnormal skin pinch, dry mucous membranes (the inner, pink part of the mouth), irritability, sunken or depressed fontanelle (in a child under 1 year), slow capillary refill (greater than 3 seconds), cold extremities, tachycardia, and hypotension. Give IV fluids and re-assess frequently. [See SKILLS]

INTRO
ABCDE
TRAUMA
BREATHING
SHOCK
AMS
SKILLS
GLOSSARY
REFS & QUICK CARDS

Malaria may be more severe in children than adults. Children with severe malaria may present with severe anaemia, seizure/convulsions, coma, and hypoglycaemia.

Ingestion of chemicals or drugs is common in children. Try to identify the poison (talk to parents) and try to get a photograph of the package. Consult advanced provider immediately for management.

Consider unwitnessed ingestions in children aged under 6 years (especially aged 1–3):

- Ask about signs and symptoms depending on the substance ingested.
- Take a thorough history from the family.
- Examine the bottles of the ingested substance or medicine.
- Determine what time it took place.
- Ensure that no other children were involved.
- Check for signs of burns in or around the mouth
- Check for stridor (high-pitched noises) suggesting ingestion of chemicals that burned or damaged the airway and are causing swelling.
- Children with ingestion of drugs or chemicals need to be monitored closely and may require handover/transfer to a referral unit for further management.

Workbook question 5: Altered mental status

Using the workbook section above, answer the following questions about altered mental status in children:

How would you assess for brain infection in a child?

_____

_____

Why does hypoglycaemia occur frequently in severely ill children?

_____

Seizures/convulsions in young children can be a sign of what?

_____

INTRO

ABCDE

TRAUMA

BREATHING

SHOCK

AMS

SKILLS

GLOSSARY

REFS & QUICK CARDS

DISPOSITION CONSIDERATIONS

Disposition depends on the cause of altered mental status. Causes of altered mental status that cannot be rapidly corrected or which might return after medications wear off need management in a hospital setting.

- Any patient with altered mental status must be closely monitored for airway problems. Consider handover/transfer to a provider with advanced airway capabilities.

- If the underlying cause of the low blood glucose is not identified and treated, patients with hypoglycaemia who improved with glucose may develop low blood glucose again and may require repeat treatments. These patients need to be monitored closely.

- Naloxone (opioid reversal agent) effects only last approximately 1 hour. Many opioid medications are longer-acting and may need more doses of naloxone to reverse the opioid effects. Any patient treated with naloxone must be monitored closely. Make sure the new provider knows the patient has been given naloxone and may need additional doses.

FACILITATOR-LED CASE SCENARIOS

These case scenarios will be presented in small groups. One participant will be identified as the lead and will be assessed, while the rest of the group writes the responses in the workbook. To complete a case scenario, the group must identify the critical findings and management needed, and formulate a one-line summary for handover, including assessment findings and interventions. You should use the Quick Card for these scenarios while being assessed.

CASE #1: ADULT WITH ALTERED MENTAL STATUS

A 42-year-old man is brought in after he was found slumped over at a bus stop. When the bystanders went to him he was awake but very confused. They do not know him, but because he is so confused they brought him to you for care.

1. **What do you need to do in your initial approach?**

2. **Use the ABCDE approach to assess and manage this patient. Ask the facilitator about look, listen and feel findings; use the Quick Card for reference as needed.**

	ASSESSMENT	FINDINGS	INTERVENTION NEEDED?		INTERVENTION TO PERFORM:
AIRWAY			YES	NO	
BREATHING			YES	NO	

	ASSESSMENT	FINDINGS	INTERVENTION NEEDED?		INTERVENTION TO PERFORM:
CIRCULATION			YES	NO	
DISABILITY			YES	NO	
EXPOSURE			YES	NO	

3. Formulate one sentence to summarize this patient for handover.

CASE #2: PAEDIATRIC PATIENT WITH ALTERED MENTAL STATUS

A mother brings her 3-year-old child to you for evaluation after she had two seizures/convulsions today. The child is wrapped in multiple blankets. The mother states that the child has been increasingly confused over the past 2 days and has had high fevers.

1. What do you need to do in your initial approach?

2. Use the ABCDE approach to assess and manage this patient. Ask the facilitator about look, listen and feel findings; use the Quick Card for reference as needed.

	ASSESSMENT	FINDINGS	INTERVENTION NEEDED?		INTERVENTION TO PERFORM:
AIRWAY			YES	NO	
BREATHING			YES	NO	
CIRCULATION			YES	NO	
DISABILITY			YES	NO	
EXPOSURE			YES	NO	

3. Formulate one sentence to summarize this patient for handover.

MULTIPLE CHOICE QUESTIONS

Answer the questions below. Questions and answers will be discussed in the session.

1. You are evaluating ABCDE on a 4-year-old boy who has a fever and a cough. He is not responding to you calling his name, but if you pinch the sole of his foot, he moans. What is his level on the AVPU scale?

   A. Alert

   B. Verbal

   C. Pain

   D. Unresponsive

2. A 37-year-old male is brought in by his wife with fever and confusion. She says since the fever began 3 days ago he has become increasingly confused. There has been no trauma. On examination you notice that his neck is stiff. What is the most likely cause of his altered mental status?

   A. Pneumonia

   B. Infection around the brain

   C. Stroke

   D. Drug use

3. A 46-year-old man comes in to check his blood pressure. His vital signs are: blood pressure 160/90, heart rate 120, respiratory rate 18, and blood glucose is 5 mmol/L. While you are examining him he has a seizure/convulsion. What treatment should you give?

   A. Benzodiazepine

   B. Glucose

   C. Antibiotics

   D. Naloxone

4. A 36-week pregnant woman is having a seizure/convulsion. She has a recent history of high blood pressure as well. What treatment should you give?

   A. Magnesium sulphate

   B. Glucose

   C. Nitroglycerin

   D. Nothing, the seizure/convulsion will stop on its own

5. You are assessing a 6-month-old infant and find a depressed fontanelle. What does this physical examination finding suggest?

   A. Infection in the brain

   B. Dehydration

   C. Pneumonia

   D. Hypoglycaemia

INTRO

ABCDE

TRAUMA

BREATHING

SHOCK

AMS

SKILLS

GLOSSARY

REFS & QUICK CARDS

Notes

WHO BASIC EMERGENCY CARE [SKILLS]

INTRO

ABCDE

TRAUMA

BREATHING

SHOCK

AMS

SKILLS

GLOSSARY

REFS & QUICK CARDS

INTRO

ABCDE

TRAUMA

BREATHING

SHOCK

AMS

SKILLS

GLOSSARY

REFS & QUICK CARDS

TABLE OF CONTENTS: SKILLS

SKILLS

SKILL STATIONS are designed to allow you to practise new skills and demonstrate life-saving techniques.

> REMEMBER...ALWAYS WEAR PROPER PPE PRIOR TO CARING FOR A PATIENT AND PERFORMING ANY SKILL.

1. AIRWAY SKILL STATIONS

AIRWAY SKILL STATION: BASIC AIRWAY MANOEUVRES

Opening the airway: adult head-tilt and chin-lift

To be used for patients with altered mental status who may not be able to protect the airway, with NO history of trauma:

- Place person face up on flat, firm surface.
- Tilt the head back with one hand and lift the chin with your fingers.
  - To do this, place one hand on the patient's forehead and then place two fingers of the other hand on the chin. Rotate your hands, tilting the chin up away from the chest.
- Remove foreign bodies if visible.
- Use suction to remove any liquids or secretions from the airway if needed.
- Hold the airway open – do not let the head drop back as this will close the airway.

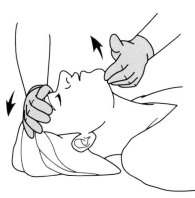

Adult head-tilt and chin lift

Opening the airway: paediatric head-tilt and chin-lift

To be used with patients with altered mental status who may not be able to protect the airway, with NO history of trauma:

- Remember, children's heads are bigger than adults' heads compared to body size, and their airways are softer and easier to block when the neck is bent. In older children, the airway can be opened by tilting the head backwards slightly (see figure).
- Babies have the largest heads relative to their body size. Their heads should be placed in neutral (sniffing) position (see figure).
- Inspect the mouth and remove visible foreign bodies. Take care not to push the foreign body deeper into the airway.

INTRO

ABCDE

TRAUMA

BREATHING

SHOCK

AMS

SKILLS

GLOSSARY

REFS & QUICK CARDS

• Use suction to remove any liquids or secretions from the airway.
• Hold the head as below in position to keep the airway open.

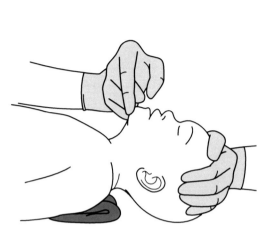

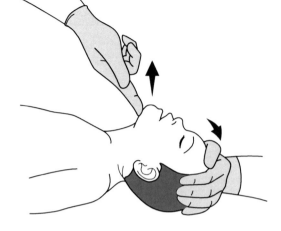

Neutral position in infants   *Head-tilt and chin-lift in children (no trauma)*

Opening the airway: adult and paediatric jaw thrust

Use when the patient has altered mental status and may not be able to protect the airway and there IS a history of trauma (cervical spine fracture is possible):

• Ask an assistant to immobilize the cervical spine while you perform the jaw thrust. [See SKILLS]
• Place fingers behind the angle of mandible (the curve on the jaw bone) on both sides of the jaw and push up so that the lower jaw moves. The head and neck should NOT move.
• Inspect the mouth and remove foreign bodies if visible.
• Use suction to remove any liquids or secretions from the airway if needed.
• Hold the jaw in place to keep the airway open – do not let the jaw drop back as this will close the airway.

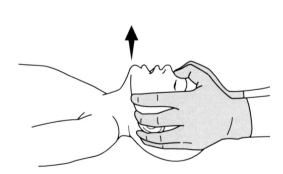

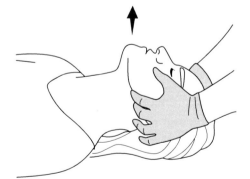

Jaw thrust in children   *Jaw thrust in adults*

AIRWAY SKILL STATION: MANAGEMENT OF CHOKING

Managing choking in an adult or larger child

If respiratory distress occurs suddenly while eating, a person is clutching the throat, or there is silent coughing, cyanosis (skin turns blue in colour), stridor or noisy breathing, suspect a foreign body obstructing the airway.

Encourage the person to speak or cough if possible and observe if the obstruction is removed. Do not perform the manoeuvres described below if the person is audibly coughing and/or able to make sounds.

A person who is unable to speak or cough has complete airway obstruction and needs immediate help:

• Tell the person that you are going to provide help.

• Deliver five abdominal thrusts (see below for modifications for pregnant women).

  – Stand behind the person and lean the person forward.

  – Form a fist with one hand and place it in the centre of the abdomen between the umbilicus (belly button) and the bottom portion of breastbone.

  – Place your other hand over your fist.

  – **NOTE**: If the patient is pregnant, place the side of your fist in the center of the chest and pull sharply inward.

  – Pull in and up five times using hard, quick thrusts. This forces the air out of the patient's lungs to try to "blow out" the obstruction.

  – If the obstruction persists, have the person bend at the waist and give five back blows (with the heel of your hand, strike the back between the shoulder blades in the direction towards the head).

  – Re-assess.

  – Repeat abdominal thrusts followed by back blows until patient speaks, coughs or becomes unconscious.

  – If the choking person becomes unconscious, lie him/her face up on a firm surface. Performing chest thrusts may relieve the obstruction. If a series of chest thrusts is not successful, continue with rescue breaths and chest compressions based on relevant CPR protocols.

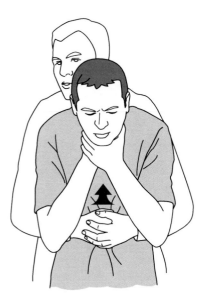

Abdominal thrusts for choking adult

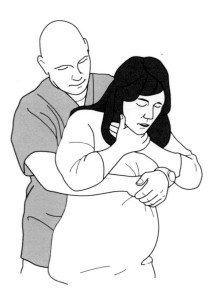

Chest thrusts for choking in late pregnancy

INTRO

ABCDE

TRAUMA

BREATHING

SHOCK

AMS

SKILLS

GLOSSARY

REFS & QUICK CARDS

Managing choking in an infant or small child

- Lay the infant on your arm or thigh in face down position with the head lower than the abdomen.
- Give five back blows (with the heel of your hand, striking the back sharply between the shoulder blades in the direction towards the head).
- If obstruction persists, turn the infant over.
- Give five chest thrust with two fingers, just below the nipple line in the midline of the chest.
- If obstruction persists, check infant's mouth for any visible obstruction that can be removed. (Caution for biting.)
- If necessary, repeat entire process until the foreign body is removed.

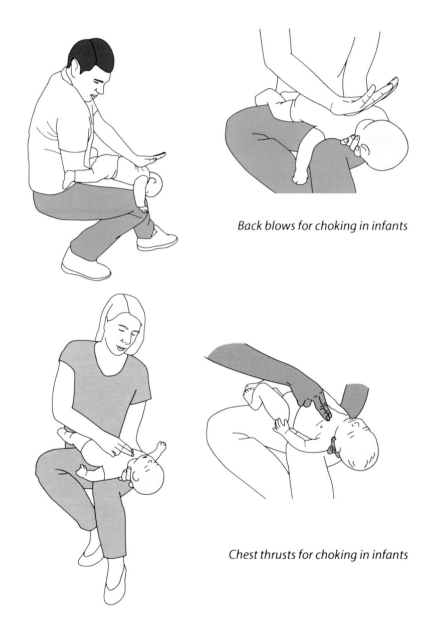

Back blows for choking in infants

Chest thrusts for choking in infants

AIRWAY SKILL STATION: AIRWAY SUCTIONING

The purpose of suctioning is to remove any liquids or secretions from the upper airway. Suctioning may be necessary to maintain an open airway if a person cannot clear secretions without help.

- Check to see if your suction canister or handheld device is working.
- Attach a rigid or soft suction catheter to the end of the suction tubing.
- Explain what you are doing.
- Insert the suction catheter into the back of the mouth (only as far back as you can see), cover the side hole on the catheter (NOT the tip of the catheter) to create suction. Suction only while pulling the catheter out and release suction when advancing the catheter forward (advancing the catheter further into the mouth while suctioning can cause injury). Repeat to suction all of the fluid in the back of the mouth.
- Do not suction for more than 10 seconds at a time unless the airway is completely blocked with fluid.
- To avoid trauma to the mouth, do not place the end of the suction tip directly against the soft tissue or hold it in just one place. Suction only in the oral cavity, do not suction up the nose.

AIRWAY SKILL STATION: BASIC AIRWAY DEVICE INSERTION

Oropharyngeal airway (OPA) insertion

- An oropharyngeal airway (OPA) should only be inserted when the person is unconscious. A conscious person will not tolerate an OPA and will push it out. If the person resists, gags or vomits, remove the device immediately.
- Always protect the cervical spine when there is a history of trauma.
- Measure the appropriate size of the OPA by measuring from the tip of the earlobe to the corner of the mouth.
- Open the person's mouth using care not to insert your fingers between the teeth (to avoid accidentally being bitten).
- Insert the OPA with the curved portion sideways and the tip pointing towards the cheek.
- Push the OPA gently into the mouth and, when you can push no further, rotate the OPA 90 degrees, so that the tip now points down the throat and follows the curve of the tongue (see figure).
- Push the OPA the remainder of the way in if necessary so that the flange (the wide, flat end) rests on the person's lips. If you have to do this, be sure that the tip of the OPA does not push the tongue down to obstruct the back of the throat.
- Check again to make sure the OPA did not push the tongue down and obstruct the airway.
- Give oxygen if available.

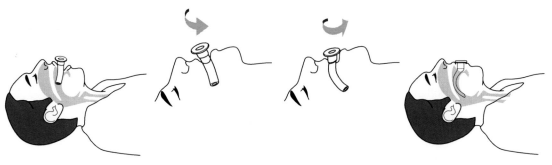

Oropharyngeal airway (OPA) insertion

INTRO

ABCDE

TRAUMA

BREATHING

SHOCK

AMS

SKILLS

GLOSSARY

REFS & QUICK CARDS

Nasopharyngeal airway (NPA) insertion

Nasopharyngeal airways (NPA) are better tolerated in people who are semi-conscious or when there is a possibility of gagging with oropharyngeal airways. DO NOT use an NPA in people with head and facial trauma.

- Assess the nasal passage for any obvious airway obstruction.
- Determine the appropriate size NPA to insert. Measure from the base of the nostrils to the earlobe. The diameter of the NPA itself needs to be smaller than the person's nasal passage.
- Lubricate the NPA well and insert it into the nostril, directing it along the floor of the nose posteriorly towards the throat until the wide, flat portion (flange) of the tube rests against the nostril.
- Give oxygen if available.

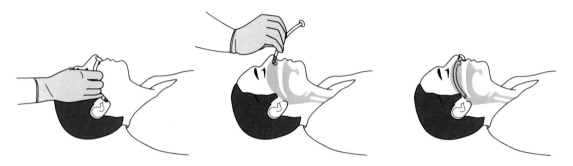

Nasopharyngeal airway (NPA) insertion

Airway skill station assessments

Skills station marking criteria	1st pass	2nd pass	3rd pass
Safety: Personal protective equipment used or verbalized.			
BASIC AIRWAY MANOEUVRES			
Skill 1 – Open the airway: head-tilt and chin-lift			
List the indications for use – non-trauma cases only.			
Tilt the head with one hand on the forehead and lift chin with fingers.			
State that a baby must be placed in a neutral (sniffing) position.			
Remove foreign bodies if visible.			
Suction airway if required.			
Hold the airway open. Do not let the head drop back as this will close the airway.			
Comments:			
Skill 2– Open the airway: jaw thrust			
List the indications for using jaw thrust versus head-tilt and chin-lift (trauma with possible cervical spine injury).			
Ask for an assistant to immobilize the cervical spine.			

INTRO

ABCDE

TRAUMA

BREATHING

SHOCK

AMS

SKILLS

GLOSSARY

REFS & QUICK CARDS

Place fingers behind the angle of mandible (the curve on the jaw bone) on both sides of the jaw and push up so that the lower jaw moves. Note that the head and neck should NOT move.

Remove any visible foreign bodies.

Hold the airway open – do not let the jaw drop back as this will close the airway.

Comments:

MANAGEMENT OF CHOKING

Skill 3 – Choking: adult and larger child

Be able to give the indication for abdominal thrusts (the person is unable to speak or cough).

Tell the person what you are going to do.

Stand behind the person and lean the person forward.

Form a fist with one hand and place it in the centre of the abdomen between the umbilicus and the bottom portion of breastbone.

Cover one fist with your other hand.

Pull in and up five times using hard quick thrusts. This forces the air out of the patient's lungs to try to "blow out" the obstruction.

Assume the victim is still choking: have the person bend at the waist.

Deliver five back blows with the heel of one hand between the shoulder blades, striking the back in the direction towards the head.

State that you will re-assess the patient

Repeat abdominal thrust then back blows until patient speaks or coughs or becomes unconscious.

State how this would be modified for a pregnant woman:

• Rather than abdominal thrust, place the side of fist in the centre of the chest, cover fist with other hand, and pull sharply inward.

Comments:

Skill 4 – Management of the choking infant and small child

Lay the infant over your arm or thigh in the face down position with the head lower than the abdomen.

Give five back blows to the infant's back between the shoulder blades with the heel of one hand.

If obstruction persists, turn the infant over.

Give five chest thrusts with two fingers placed just below the nipple line in the middle of the chest.

If obstruction persists, check infant's mouth for any obstruction that can be removed.

Repeat until obstruction is removed.

Comments:

Skill 5 – Suctioning the airway

Check your suction canister or handheld device to make sure it is working.

Attach a hard (yankauer) or soft suction catheter to the end of the suction tubing.

Tell the person what you are doing.

Insert the suction catheter into the back of the mouth (ONLY as far back as you can see) and cover the side hole on the catheter (NOT the tip of the catheter). Do not suction while inserting the catheter into the mouth. Suction only while pulling catheter out.

State how long the patient should be suctioned for (no more than 10 seconds at a time unless the airway is completely covered with fluid).

State the need to constantly move the suction catheter and not put the suction tip against the soft tissue.

Comments:

BASIC AIRWAY DEVICE INSERTION

Skill 6 – Oropharyngeal airway (OPA)

List the indication for using an oropharyngeal airway (person is unconscious with no gag reflex).

Determine the appropriate size OPA to insert: (participant should explain how to do this out loud).
• Measure from the earlobe to the corner of the mouth on that side.

Open the mouth using care not to insert your fingers between the teeth (to avoid accidentally being bitten).

Insert the OPA with the curved portion sideways and the tip pointing to the cheek.

Once the OPA is in as a far as it will go, rotate the oropharyngeal 90 degrees so that the tip now points down the throat and the curve follows the tongue.

Push the OPA the remainder of the way in so that the flange (the flat end) rests on the person's lips.

Check to make sure the OPA did not push the tongue down to obstruct the airway.

State that oxygen will be given if available.

Comments:

Skill 7 – Nasopharyngeal Airway (NPA)

List the indications for an NPA. (Better tolerated in a person who is semi-conscious or who may still have a gag reflex).

State that NPAs should not be used in people with head and facial trauma.

Assess the nasal passage for any obvious airway obstruction.

Explain how to determine the appropriate size NPA to insert:
- Measure from the external portion of the nostril to the bottom of the earlobe.
- The diameter of the tube should not be bigger than the nostril (nasal passage).

Lubricate the NPA.

Lift up the tip of the nose.

Insert the lubricated NPA into the nostril and gently push it along the floor of the nose until the flared-out base (flange) rests against the nostril.

State that oxygen will be given if available.

Comments:

Competency demonstrated	YES	NO
Remediation required	YES	NO
Signature of facilitator:		

INTRO
ABCDE
TRAUMA
BREATHING
SHOCK
AMS
SKILLS
GLOSSARY
REFS & QUICK CARDS

2. BREATHING SKILL STATIONS

BREATHING SKILL STATION: BREATHING EXAM

- Assess and count the rate of breathing (normal is between 10–20 breaths per minute in an adult. See ABCDE module for normal paediatric values).
- Look for increased work of breathing (nasal flaring, retractions or chest in-drawing).
- Feel for chest rise and chest wall tenderness.
- Percuss the chest wall:
  - Place one hand on the chest with fingers separated (the middle finger should lie between the ribs).
  - With the other hand, tap on the middle finger of the first hand and listen for changes in tone (hollow or dull).
- Listen to the chest:
  - Always expose the chest. Never listen through clothes.
  - Make sure your stethoscope is not too cold.
  - Place your stethoscope lightly on the chest wall. Ask the patient to open his or her mouth and take a complete deep breath in and out. Listen to the sounds of the breathing and compare the left side to the right. Listen in the upper zone, middle zone and lower zones and listen to the front of the chest and the back.
  - Normal breath sounds like wind moving in and out, while abnormal breathing sounds like air going through water, crumpling paper bags, or no air moving at all. [See DIB]
  - Respect modesty and avoid placing the stethoscope directly on the breasts when possible.

BREATHING SKILL STATION: GIVING SUPPLEMENTAL OXYGEN

Supplemental oxygen should be given when the patient has signs and symptoms of hypoxia – fast breathing, anxiety, excessive sweating, cyanosis or chest pain. Where available, a pulse oximeter should be used to measure oxygen saturation.

- If hypoxia does not appear severe, lower levels of oxygen (24–40% oxygen) can be provided to children and adults through **nasal cannula** (nasal prongs), but monitor closely in case a mask is needed. (*Remember*, regular air is approximately 21% oxygen)
  - Nasal cannula should be about half the size of the nostril.
  - Position the cannula in each nostril, making sure that it does not extend too far back or press on the tissues.
  - Secure the tubing to the cheeks or loop the tubing over the ears so that the nasal prongs and the tubing are both on the front side of the patient's body (never put the head through the loop in the tubing – if patients become confused and hypoxic, they can accidentally strangle themselves).
  - Oxygen is delivered at a low rate: max 5 L/min.
- If hypoxia appears more severe (or if signs of hypoxia continue with maximum oxygen flow via nasal cannula), a simple facemask may be used. Simple facemask is usually used with oxygen flow rates of 6–10 L/min and can deliver approximately 40–60% oxygen.
  - The facemask is applied to the face, ensuring the bridge of the nose is covered and as little as possible leaks along the side. The mask should rest below the lower lip, but not past the chin. The elastic strap should be placed over the head to secure the mask.
- For patients who appear extremely hypoxic or who still have signs of hypoxia with a simple facemask, oxygen can be delivered through a **non-rebreather facemask**. This provides close to 100% oxygen if the reservoir bag is full.
  - To prepare the non-rebreather facemask, put one finger over the valve at the top of the reservoir bag inside the mask to inflate the bag. Then apply the non-rebreather facemask in the same way as the simple facemask, ensuring as little leakage as possible.
  - Make sure that the oxygen is attached to the wall or cannister and that the flow rate is between 10–15 L/min depending on the pressure in your oxygen system and how fast and deep the patient breathes. If the patient is still hypoxic or the non-rebreather facemask bag does not fill, increase the oxygen flow rate.

– NEVER put a non-rebreather facemask on before it is connected to oxygen. A true non-rebreather mask will not allow outside air in and can worsen difficulty in breathing and hypoxia if there is no oxygen flowing through the tubing.

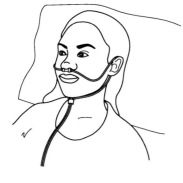

Nasal cannula/prongs

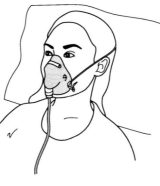

Simple facemask

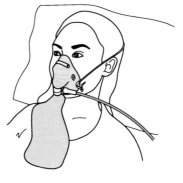

Non-rebreather

BREATHING SKILL STATION: BAG-VALVE-MASK VENTILATION

Assess and manage airway and provide bag-mask-ventilation (BVM) for any patient who is not breathing or not breathing adequately (too slow for age or too shallow), any unconscious patient with abnormal breathing (slow, shallow, gasping or noisy), or any patient with a pulse who is not breathing (for patients without a pulse, follow relevant CPR protocols).

> **CAUTION!** Avoid over-aggressive ventilation (using bag-valve-mask too fast or with too much pressure) as this will damage the lungs. Children have smaller lungs that are especially fragile. When ventilating a child, be particularly careful to only give enough pressure to make the chest rise and be sure to allow enough time between breaths for exhalation (for the air to escape). Large volumes of air or high pressures may result in pneumothorax or irreversible lung damage.

Bag-mask-ventilation steps:

• If you have oxygen available, attach the BVM tubing and set the flow to the highest rate available. DO NOT DELAY bag-mask-ventilation to prepare oxygen. (Oxygen can be attached later.)

• Place the mask over the patient's mouth and nose (if you have two people available one person squeezes the bag and other holds the mask on the patient's face and keeps the airway open).

• Create a seal so that air does not leak out. Put your hand or hands in the "EC" position – your thumb and first finger should make a "C" around the top of the mask and push down evenly, your last three fingers should reach just under the bony part of the jaw (looking like an "E") and pull the jaw upward to open the airway.

– Think about pulling the face up to the mask (thus opening the airway) and pushing the mask down onto the face (creating a seal).

– If you push down too hard without pulling the face up to the mask, you will block the airway and the patient will be difficult to bag. If you have problems ventilating, reposition your hands and the mask and try again.

• If the patient is breathing on his or her own, deliver breaths when the patient takes a breath (during inspiration). Do not attempt to deliver a breath as the patient exhales.

• If you are still unable to ventilate the person after repositioning the mask, consider the possibility of foreign body obstruction or air leak. Insert an oral or nasopharyngeal airway device if not already in place (See SKILLS).

INTRO
ABCDE
TRAUMA
BREATHING
SHOCK
AMS
SKILLS
GLOSSARY
REFS & QUICK CARDS

- Hold the bag in one hand and depress the bag enough to make the chest rise (to about one third of its volume for an adult – make sure you are using the appropriate-sized bag: an adult bag should have a volume of about 2 litres).
- Squeeze bag over 1–2 seconds to provide chest rise (giving the breath faster can cause lung damage).
- Give one breath every 6 seconds (10 breaths per minute) in an adult; one breath every 4 seconds (15 breaths per minute) in older children; or one breath every 3 seconds (20 breaths per minute) in infants. CAUTION with volume of breaths given in small children (see SKILLS). Giving large volume breaths can cause pneumothorax.
- After each breath allow the chest to fall before giving another breath.
- Watch the chest rising and falling evenly with each breath.

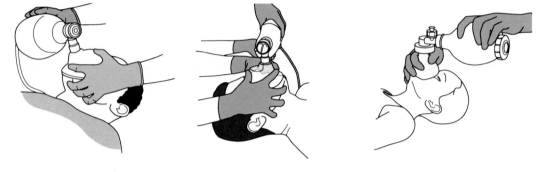

BVM: One provider   *BVM: Two providers*   *BVM: Child*

BREATHING SKILL STATION: EMERGENCY NEEDLE DECOMPRESSION

Needle decompression of the chest is a life-saving emergency procedure for suspected tension pneumothorax (presence of air or gas in the cavity between the lungs and the chest wall causing excessive pressure on the opposite lung, the great vessels, and the heart). Patients can die very quickly from a tension pneumothorax. These patients need an emergent chest tube, but emergency needle decompression will relieve the immediate pressure and allow time for handover/transfer for chest tube. **Emergency needle decompression should only be performed for tension pneumothorax.**

- Expose the chest and assess breathing.
- A tension pneumothorax is identified if shock and the following are present:
  – Difficulty in breathing
  – Absence of lung sounds on the affected side
  – Hypotension
  – Distended neck veins
  – Hyperresonance with percussion on the affected side
  – Tracheal shift away from affected side
- Insert a large-bore (14–16G preferred) IV cannula along the upper edge of the third rib through the second rib (intercostal) space in line with the midpoint of the clavicle on the affected side.
  – In tension pneumothorax, there will be a gush of expelled air
- Give oxygen at high concentration (non-rebreather mask).
- Start IV lines and give IV fluids.
- Refer and transport to definitive care immediately.

Chest tube should be placed as soon as possible following needle decompression (even if there was no rush of air) or for any suspected haemothorax.

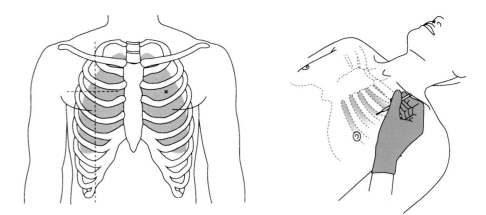

Needle decompression

BREATHING SKILL STATION: MANAGEMENT OF OPEN PNEUMOTHORAX (SUCKING CHEST WOUND)

An **open pneumothorax** is an open chest wall wound that sucks air in when the patient breathes in. Normally, when the chest wall is expanded, air is drawn into the lungs through the airway (through a vacuum effect). If there is another hole in the chest wall (due to trauma) air will also be drawn in that hole, but, rather than going into the lungs, it goes into the space between the chest wall and lungs, creating a pneumothorax. A 3-sided dressing is placed to prevent more air from coming in during inhalation, but to allow air from the pneumothorax to escape during exhalation to avoid developing a tension pneumothorax. To manage a sucking chest wound (open pneumothorax):

- Give high flow oxygen.
- Cover the sucking chest wound with petroleum gauze or other non-adhesive dressing such as the plastic wrapper from gauze packaging.
- Tape three sides of the dressing, leaving one side un-taped to act as a flap valve.
- These patients need to be transferred as soon as possible to a centre where a chest tube can be placed. (**DO NOT place a chest tube through the injury.**)

Caution! There is a danger of the dressing becoming stuck to the chest wall with clotted blood. When this happens, air cannot escape from the chest cavity and pressure can build up, leading to a tension pneumothorax. **Remove the dressing completely if there is worsening respiratory status or evidence of worsening perfusion. If the patient cannot be observed continuously, a three-sided dressing should NOT be placed.**

INTRO

ABCDE

TRAUMA

BREATHING

SHOCK

AMS

SKILLS

GLOSSARY

REFS & QUICK CARDS

BREATHING SKILL STATION: HOW TO MAKE A SPACER FROM A PLASTIC BOTTLE

The purpose of a spacer is to hold the medication (salbutamol) released from a metered dose inhaler so the person has time to effectively inhale the medication. (Without experience and proper training, it can be difficult to use a metered dose inhaler effectively and medication is often lost into the mouth or throat). Spacers should be made in advance, however. Do not delay salbutamol delivery to make a spacer.

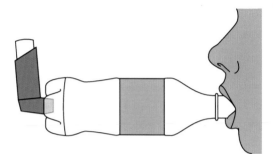

Spacer made from a plastic bottle

- Use a clean 300–500ml plastic bottle (wash with detergent and rinse and dry well).
- Take the cap off the metered dose inhaler and trace the shape of the opening of the inhaler on the base of the bottle directly opposite the mouth of the bottle.
- Cut an opening into the base of the bottle slightly smaller than the traced shape. You can cut this with scissors or a heated paper clip.
- Insert the inhaler into the spacer to check the size (the inhaler should fit tightly into the cut opening).
- Always remember to prime the spacer with five puffs before use to clear the dead space.

Breathing skill station assessments

Skills station marking criteria	1st pass	2nd pass	3rd pass
Safety: Personal protective equipment used or verbalized use.			
Skill 1– Assess breathing			
Assess and count rate of breathing.			
Look for increased work of breathing (nasal flaring, retractions).			
Feel for chest rise and chest wall tenderness.			
Percuss the chest wall.			
Listen to the chest (auscultate).			
Comments:			
Skill 2 – Supplemental oxygen administration			
State the indication for oxygen (hypoxia, indicated by fast breathing, anxiety, excess sweating, cyanosis (blue tinted skin), or chest pain).			

INTRO

ABCDE

TRAUMA

BREATHING

SHOCK

AMS

SKILLS

GLOSSARY

REFS & QUICK CARDS

Explain when **nasal cannula** should be used (mild hypoxia).

Demonstrate applying a nasal cannula with a nasal prong in each nostril.

Secure the tubing to the cheek or loop over the patient's ears. (The participant should NOT put the patient's head through the loop in the tubing.)

State that the oxygen flow rate should be no more than 5 l/min.

If the patient still has signs of hypoxia, explain which oxygen delivery method should be used next. (**Simple facemask**)

Apply **simple facemask** – mask over nose bridge and below lower lip.

Ensure minimal air leak – adjust elastic to hold in place.

Explain that the oxygen flow rate should be between 6–10 L/min.

If the patient still has signs of hypoxia, explain which oxygen delivery method should be used next. (**Non-rebreather facemask**)

To prepare the non-rebreather facemask, put one finger over the valve at the top of the reservoir bag inside the mask to inflate the bag. Ensure that the bag is inflated.

Apply **non-rebreather** facemask – mask over nose bridge and below lower lip.

Ensure minimal air leak – adjust elastic to hold in place.

Turn on oxygen to 10–15 L/min depending on patient's breathing.

Adjust non-rebreather mask, and adjust flow to ensure bag is filled partially.

Comments:

Skill 3 – Bag-valve-mask ventilation

State the indication for bag-valve-mask ventilation.

State that if oxygen is available, connect it to the bag – but do not delay BVM to prepare oxygen.

Ensure adequate mask-face seal.

State correct rate of ventilation.

State relevant cautions when ventilating a child.

Verbalize that over-aggressive ventilation can damage lungs and cause vomiting.

State or demonstrate correct volume of ventilation.

Assess chest rise.

If no chest rise, reposition airway. Consider OPA or NPA.

Comments:

Skill 4 – Emergency needle decompression

State the indication for this procedure.

Explain procedure to patient.

Expose the chest and clean the skin.

Identify landmark: second intercostal space (between the 2nd and 3rd ribs) in the midclavicular line.

Insert 14–16G IV cannula into the identified location.

Slide cannula over needle, and remove needle.

State plan to handover/transfer for chest tube

Give oxygen and assess respiratory rate, vital signs and oxygen saturation (if available).

Start IV line and give IV fluids.

Comments:

Skill 5 – Management of open pneumothorax (sucking chest wound)

Give high flow oxygen.

Cover with petroleum gauze.

Tape 3 sides of gauze.

State the need for a chest tube to be inserted.

Describe the risk of a clotted dressing blocking outflow of air.

Comments:

Competency demonstrated	YES	NO
Remediation required	YES	NO
Signature of Facilitator:		

3. CIRCULATION SKILL STATIONS

CIRCULATION SKILL STATION: CIRCULATION EXAM

- Check for anxiety, confusion or altered mental status.
- Feel for a pulse, assessing rate and quality (normal range is 60–100 beats per minute in adults. See ABCDE for normal paediatric values).
- Assess capillary refill (checked by pushing on the fingernail, palms, or soles and releasing to see how long it takes for the colour to return to the skin). The normal range is less than 3 seconds.
- Assess the skin colour and touch the skin to assess the temperature.
- Measure other vital signs: respiratory rate and blood pressure (normal adult values: RR 10–20 breaths per minute and systolic BP greater than 90 mmHG. See ABCDE for normal paediatric values).

CIRCULATION SKILL STATION EXAM: EXTERNAL BLEEDING CONTROL

Direct pressure for external bleeding

A wound that is deep and bleeding heavily may not stop bleeding on its own. Applying direct pressure with a clean dressing such as gauze can help to slow or stop the bleeding (see figure).

- Put on gloves.
- Use gauze or another clean non-adherent dressing.
- Do not use bulky dressings as they can make it difficult to put enough pressure in the right place.
- Apply firm pressure as directly as possible to the source of bleeding, usually with two or three fingers.
- If the wound is on a limb, elevate the limb above the heart.
- If the first dressing becomes soaked with blood, do not remove as this will dislodge any clots that have formed. Instead add another pad and apply firm pressure.
- When bleeding stops, apply a bandage to keep the gauze/pad in place.
- If bleeding does not stop, consider deep wound packing or tourniquet (see next section).

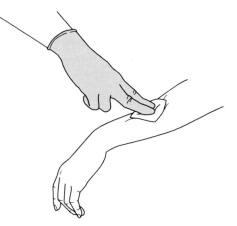

Applying direct pressure to a wound

INTRO
ABCDE
TRAUMA
BREATHING
SHOCK
AMS
SKILLS
GLOSSARY
REFS & QUICK CARDS

Deep wound packing for external bleeding

If the wound is deep or gaping and simple pressure does not stop the bleeding, deep wound packing may help. However, deep wound packing is a **temporary** procedure to stop the bleeding since it can lead to infection if left for more than 24 hours.

- Put on gloves.
- Always assess pulses, capillary refill and sensation **before and after** dressing or splinting any wound.
- Thoroughly wash out the wound by flushing with at least a litre of clean water (under pressure when possible; see next section).
- Use gauze or another clean, compact material to completely fill the space within the wound.
- Use additional gauze on top of the wound surface and apply direct pressure with your gloved hand or a bandage wrapped firmly around the wound/limb.
- For limb wounds requiring packing, apply a splint to reduce the risk of re-bleeding.
- A deep wound pack should not be left in place for more than 24 hours because of the risk of infection.
- If bleeding does not stop, consider tourniquet (see next section).

Tourniquet technique for uncontrolled external bleeding

You will not be expected to perform the tourniquet technique BUT you will be expected to know what life-threatening conditions it can be used for, the special considerations around use of a tourniquet and the ongoing care of the patient.

Use this technique **ONLY** if all other bleeding control measures have failed **AND** haemorrhage is **life-threatening.** If you place a tourniquet, there is a possibility that tissues below the tourniquet will be permanently damaged and even require amputation. If you are considering using a tourniquet, **CALL FOR HELP IMMEDIATELY** and plan for handover/transfer to a unit where surgery is possible.

- If available, use a pneumatic tourniquet (like a blood pressure cuff) over padded skin and inflate until bleeding stops. If not, use a thick band or piece of cloth or belt (the wider, the better), over padded skin.
- Apply as close to wound as possible, but do not place over a wound or a fracture.
- Apply enough pressure to make distal pulses disappear and re-assess bleeding.
- If bleeding stops, leave dressing in place if already present or dress the wound and prepare for handover/transfer to a surgical care unit.
- If the bleeding does not stop, increase tourniquet pressure until major bleeding ceases.
- Record the exact time the tourniquet was applied in the notes AND write it on the patient's skin or the tourniquet itself.
- Consult advanced provider as soon as possible (and never more than 2 hours) after placing a tourniquet.
- The tourniquet should be released every 2 hours for at least 10 minutes. Hold direct pressure to the bleeding area during this time. Do not re-apply the tourniquet unless evidence of continued active bleeding.
- Location of the tourniquet: tourniquets should only be placed on extremities and should be placed above the level of the bleeding. Because of the relationship between the bones and blood vessels, tourniquets on the upper arm or leg are often more effective than tourniquets placed below the elbow or knee.
- Make sure the tourniquet is clearly visible.
- Remember tourniquet should be placed as a last resort. If you place a tourniquet, you are cutting off blood supply to the limb, so only do this for life-threatening bleeding. When tourniquet use is absolutely necessary, use a wide, yet constrictive, band.

PARTICIPANT WORKBOOK

INTRO

ABCDE

TRAUMA

BREATHING

SHOCK

AMS

SKILLS

GLOSSARY

REFS & QUICK CARDS

CIRCULATION SKILL: UTERINE MASSAGE FOR POSTPARTUM HAEMORRHAGE

Some bleeding will occur with every delivery. After delivery, the uterus should contract, which compresses vessels and limits bleeding. Failure of the uterus to contract is the top cause of abnormal bleeding after delivery (postpartum haemorrhage). Call for help, arrange for rapid handover/transfer, start uterine massage and give oxytocin immediately.

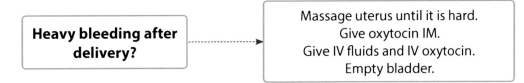

Postpartum Haemorrhage

1. Arrange immediate transfer to qualified obstetric provider!

2. Attempt to control bleeding while arranging and during transfer.

| Heavy bleeding after delivery? | ----→ | Massage uterus until it is hard.
Give oxytocin IM.
Give IV fluids and IV oxytocin.
Empty bladder. |

3. Check:

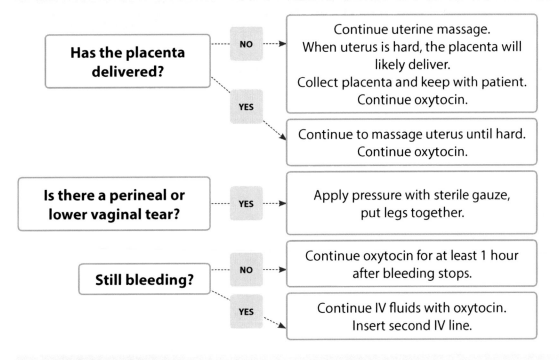

Has the placenta delivered?	NO →	Continue uterine massage. When uterus is hard, the placenta will likely deliver. Collect placenta and keep with patient. Continue oxytocin.
	YES →	Continue to massage uterus until hard. Continue oxytocin.
Is there a perineal or lower vaginal tear?	YES →	Apply pressure with sterile gauze, put legs together.
Still bleeding?	NO →	Continue oxytocin for at least 1 hour after bleeding stops.
	YES →	Continue IV fluids with oxytocin. Insert second IV line.

4. Transfer immediately

Performing uterine massage for postpartum haemorrhage

- Explain to the woman what you will do and why.
- The goal is to compress the uterus between your hand and bony structures behind the uterus (e.g. sacrum/lower back).
- Place your hand on the woman's abdomen. Through the abdominal wall, feel for the uterus and cup it with your hand. This will ensure it stays under your hand whilst you are massaging it. Do not simply squeeze the uterus, but ensure that you are applying strong pressure toward the patient's back while massaging with a circular motion.
- Massage the uterus until it is very firm. It should feel like a 10 cm rock in the lower abdomen when contracted.
- Do not stop massaging until the uterus is contracted (hard).
- Make sure the uterus does not become relaxed (soft) after you stop uterine massage. If it becomes relaxed, resume massage.
- Continuously re-assess for vaginal bleeding.
- Perform frequent vital signs.

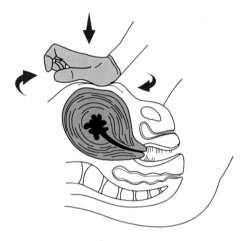

Uterine massage for postpartum hemorrhage

CIRCULATION SKILL: IV CANNULATION

Insertion of IV cannula (adult)

Inserting an IV cannula is an essential skill required for the treatment of shock. If an adult displays any signs and symptoms of shock, insert two large-bore cannulae (14 or 16 gauge).

- Prepare cannula, IV fluid of choice, tourniquet, gloves, dressing to cover the cannula and alcohol swab.
- Put on gloves.
- Place an elastic band or glove around the arm to function as a temporary tourniquet to help the veins engorge (this "tourniquet" is different from the one above and should not be so tight as to cut off arterial blood flow). Avoid placing an IV in any arm that might have a fistula for treatment of kidney disease.
- Look and feel for a vein that is straight. Avoid blood vessels that have a pulse. If a person is in shock, it may be difficult to find a vein. In this case search for a vein in the antecubital fossa (where the elbow bends, see figure).

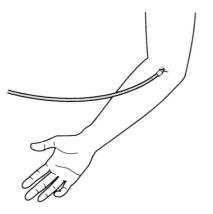

IV in antecubital fossa

- Use alcohol or other appropriate skin cleanser to wipe the skin around the vein you plan to use.
- DO NOT insert an IV through skin that is broken or appears infected.
- Prepare the cannula. Preparation may vary depending on local resources and types of cannula.
- Tell the patient what you are doing.
- Remove the safety covering over the cannula (the only thing that should be inserted is the needle with overlying plastic cannula).
- Insert the needle directly over and in line with the vein as flat and parallel to the skin as possible. Watch for flashback (flash of blood in the cannula) when you enter the vein.
  – If blood has a regular pumping pattern, you have likely hit an artery and you should remove the needle/catheter and apply firm pressure to the site for at least 5–10 minutes.
- After seeing the flash of blood, insert the needle a few millimeters further, then advance the plastic cannula over the needle fully into the patient's vein. (Do NOT let the needle move forward when you start to move the plastic cannula.)
- Hold the cannula in place, applying pressure to the base of the cannula (to occlude it and stop the flow of blood) and withdraw the needle, leaving the cannula positioned in the vein. If needed, withdraw blood to send for laboratory testing.
- Remove the IV tourniquet and flush the cannula with normal saline.
- Place a cap on the end of the cannula, secure the cannula well and dress the site. Document the date the cannula was inserted in the notes.
- Ensure the needle is placed into a sharps container.

Check IV site daily for signs of infections such as skin redness, pain and swelling. Ensure the cannula is still in the vein and not sitting in the skin next to the vein allowing fluid to be infused under the skin creating pain and swelling. If any sign of swelling or infection, remove the IV cannula and re-assess.

INTRO

ABCDE

TRAUMA

BREATHING

SHOCK

AMS

SKILLS

GLOSSARY

REFS & QUICK CARDS

Insertion of IV cannula (paediatric)

Attempt to place the cannula in the hand of the child first.

Other sites that can be used to insert a cannula include:

- Scalp veins
- External jugular veins
- Antecubital veins
- Femoral veins

When preparing for IV cannulation in children ask another assistant or parent to help keep the child's arm still.

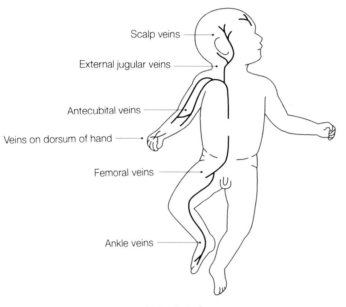

Veins in infants

- Prepare a 21 or 23 gauge cannula.
- When inserting the cannula into the back of the hand, keep the hand bent to obstruct venous return and make the veins visible. Place an "IV tourniquet" (as above) if needed. If you use an IV tourniquet, be sure you don't forget to remove it.
- Insert the cannula using the same technique used in adults. Again, be sure that the blood flows smoothly from the catheter and is not pumping. After insertion, withdraw blood if required for laboratory investigation. Remove the tourniquet and flush the cannula with a small amount of normal saline after insertion.
- Secure the cannula well. Children will attempt to remove the cannula and will undo dressings. Avoid placing a single piece of tape (plaster) that goes all the way around an extremity as this may limit blood flow.
- If the IV is placed near a joint (hand, antecubital fossa, femoral area) splint the joint to stop it from bending and preventing the IV fluid flowing in, and lightly bandage the IV site with bulky dressings to prevent the child from pulling at the adhesive dressing underneath.

INTRO

ABCDE

TRAUMA

BREATHING

SHOCK

AMS

SKILLS

GLOSSARY

REFS & QUICK CARDS

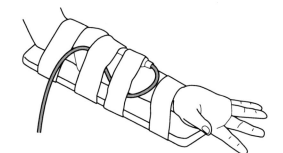

Securing an IV in a child

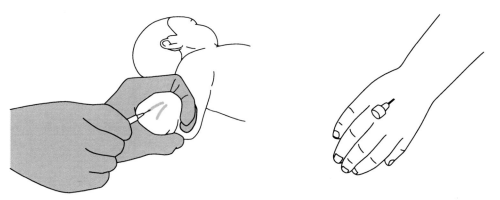

Inserting IV in a small child's hand

Check IV site daily for signs of infections such as skin redness, pain and swelling. Ensure the cannula is still in the vein and not sitting in the skin next to the vein allowing fluid to be infused into the skin creating pain, swelling and another source of infection. If any sign of infection, remove the IV cannula and re-assess.

CIRCULATION SKILL: IV FLUID – ADJUSTING FLUID VOLUME FOR SPECIAL CONDITIONS

Shock should be treated with IV fluids. Fluid volume must be adjusted for patients with three conditions: **malnutrition**, **severe anaemia** and **fluid overload**. When administering IV fluid to any patient, look for signs of new or worsening **fluid overload**: difficulty in breathing, crackles in the lungs, increasing respiratory rate or increasing heart rate. Stop IV fluids if there are any of these signs and plan for immediate handover to an advanced provider.

Recognizing conditions needing IV fluid adjustment in patients with shock – fluid overload, malnutrition, and severe anaemia.

1. Is there fluid overload?

In some patients, such as those with heart or kidney failure, there may be extra fluid in the tissues (for example, in the lungs or the soft tissues of the legs). These patients can be fluid "overloaded" even when they have poor perfusion (because the extra fluid is not in the blood vessels). These patients still need IV fluid if they are in shock, but IV fluid must be given more slowly with careful monitoring so that the fluid overload does not get worse.

CHECK FOR: Signs of fluid overload.

- Difficulty in breathing with crackles on chest exam
- Lower body swelling (usually in the legs)
- Unable to lie flat
- Distended neck veins
    - **If signs of fluid overload are present, you must adjust fluids:**
        - **Small amount** of fluids may be given (250–500 ml boluses in adults).
        - **Slow the rate** of fluid administration.
        - **Monitor closely** for worsening signs of fluid overload (increasing respiratory rate or heart rate, new or worsening difficulty breathing and increasing crackles in the chest).
        - **Stop IV fluids** if any of these signs develop.
        - **REMEMBER:** It is important to go slowly so you can stop for early signs of fluid overload. If you don't stop IV fluid when these early signs develop, too much IV fluid can cause a patient's lungs to fill with fluid and create severe difficulty in breathing, or even death.

2. Does the patient have severe anaemia?

In patients with severe anaemia, IV fluid can dilute the blood and lower its capacity to carry oxygen to dangerous levels. Additionally, patients with severe anaemia tend to show signs of fluid overload more quickly with IV fluid administration. *Remember:* you should only give IV fluids to someone with severe anaemia if there are signs of shock (see figure).

CHECK FOR: Signs of severe anaemia.

- Severe pallor to the palms of the hands (compare to your own palm) or the mucous membranes.
- Fast breathing or fast heart rate
- Confusion or restlessness
- May also have signs of heart failure/fluid overload
- **If these signs of severe anaemia are present, you must adjust fluids:**
    - **Slow the rate** of fluid administration.
    - **Monitor closely** and stop IV fluids for worsening.
    - Rapid handover/transfer to a centre capable of blood transfusion.

3. Is the patient severely malnourished?

- IV fluid can cause life-threatening swelling and heart failure in malnourished patients and must be adjusted very carefully. Malnourished patients are also at very high risk of hypoglycaemia.

CHECK FOR: Signs of malnourishment.

- Visible wasting: a child with severe wasting does not look just thin, but is visibly bony with skin that appears too large for the body. The arms, legs and buttocks may be thin, and the head may appear relatively large because of wasting of the body.
- Oedema of both feet: take shoes or socks off and assess both feet for oedema. Press the top of the foot gently with your thumb for a few seconds to see if a dent remains in the tissues. Remember that a severely malnourished child may not appear very thin if there is a lot of oedema.
  - **If these signs of severe malnutrition are present, you must adjust fluids.** [See FLUID ADMINISTRATION IN SHOCK (CHILD WITH SEVERE MALNUTRITION) for detailed fluid choice and administration rates]
    - **Oral fluid is preferred** if the patient can tolerate it.
    - **Add dextrose:** use dextrose-containing fluids or give a dose of dextrose with IV fluids.
    - **Slow the rate** of fluid administration.
    - **Monitor closely** and stop IV fluids for any signs of fluid overload.
    - **Switch** to oral fluid as soon as possible.

Visible severe wasting in a child:	Assessing for bilateral oedema in severe malnutrition in children:
• Skin looks too large for the body • There is no fat on the child • Outlines of ribs can be seen • Severe muscle wasting of the arms, legs and buttocks • The head may appear relatively large because of wasting of the body (see figure)	• Use your thumb to press gently for a few seconds on the top of each foot – the child has oedema if there is an impression when you lift your thumb • Repeat on the other foot (see figure)

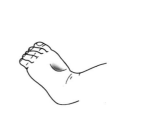

Assessing for pitting edema in children with malnutrition

Visible severe wasting in a child

INTRO
ABCDE
TRAUMA
BREATHING
SHOCK
AMS
SKILLS
GLOSSARY
REFS & QUICK CARDS

CIRCULATION SKILL: IV FLUID – ADMINISTRATION

Fluid administration for shock in adults

- Attach normal saline or Lactated Ringer's solution to the cannula.
- In adults give **1 litre** over less than 30 minutes.
- Assess response to fluid immediately after the fluid bolus. Assess perfusion (capillary refill, mental status, urine output), and check for pulse rate and blood pressure. If improving, the pulse rate should lower and the blood pressure should increase. Mental status may also improve.
- Assess for fluid overload (see signs above).
- If still in shock with no evidence of fluid overload, give another **1 litre bolus**.
- If still in shock after **2 litres of IV fluid**, re-assess for ongoing blood loss (external and internal) or spinal injury, and call for advanced provider.

If there is evidence of severe malnutrition, severe anaemia or fluid overload:

- Patients with shock still need IV fluids, but it is important to re-assess frequently for signs of worsening overload.
  - For these adult patients who are at high risk for fluid overload, bolus with 500 ml IV fluid initially, then re-assess. If no signs of fluid overload or fluid in the lungs, give additional 500 ml.

Fluid administration for shock in children

The appropriate amount of fluid for critically ill children is controversial given recent evidence that bolus fluids can worsen outcomes in some children. In addition, relevant criteria for poor perfusion and shock may vary by context. The 2016 WHO guidelines for the care of critically ill children (see WHO Sources section) use the presence of three clinical features to define shock requiring bolus fluids: cold extremities, capillary refill greater than 3 seconds, and weak and fast pulse.

For children with poor perfusion that is due to loss of fluid, such as those with bleeding, burns or severe diarrhoea/vomiting, bolus fluids are also recommended.

For other children with evidence of poor perfusion, smaller amounts of fluids given more slowly may be safer.

Country teams should consider the clinical presentation of the child, the capacity of providers to detect signs of fluid overload, and the availability of monitoring and support equipment when adapting recommendations to the national context.

To give IV fluid resuscitation to a child in shock WITHOUT severe malnutrition, severe anaemia or overload:

- Insert IV cannula as described above.
- Weigh the child or ask the parents for a recent weight.
- Give normal saline or Lactated Ringer's: 10–20 ml per kilogram of body weight over 30 minutes.

Re-assess the child after the first infusion.

- If no improvement, repeat 10 ml per kilogram of body weight over 30 minutes.

Call for help and plan to handover to an advanced provider and unit with the capacity for blood transfusion.

IV fluid resuscitation for a child in shock WITH severe malnutrition

Children that are in shock AND have severe malnutrition require specialized fluids (if available) with different rates of infusion. Children with severe malnutrition and shock are at very high risk of hypoglycaemia and will need sugar in addition to fluids. [See MEDICATIONS] If the child can take oral fluids, give oral rehydration with ReSoMal (unless the child is in shock due to cholera, then use ORS). If the child is lethargic, unconscious or not capable of taking oral fluids, then give IV fluids.

> **CAUTION!** Intravenous fluid administration can be dangerous in malnourished children. While giving fluid in any way, you must check every 5 minutes for the following danger signs: new or worsening DIB, respiratory rate increase of >5 per minute or heart rate increase of >15 beats per minute. Stop fluids if any danger sign develops.

- Insert IV line as above.
- Weigh the child.
- Give 10–15 ml per kilogram of IV fluid over 1 hour. If specialized fluids are available, give one of the following according to availability:
  - Ringer's Lactate with 5% glucose (dextrose)
  - Half-strength Darrow's solution with 5% glucose (dextrose)
  - 0.45% normal saline with 5% glucose (dextrose).
- If you do not have dextrose-containing fluids, then give one of the following:
  - Ringer's Lactate **AND** give a separate oral or IV dose of dextrose [See MEDICATIONS]
  - Normal saline **AND** give a separate oral or IV dose of dextrose. [See MEDICATIONS]

Re-assess the child after the first 5–10 minutes of the infusion and then every 5 minutes:

If the child worsens during rehydration (increased difficulty in breathing, breathing rate increases by 5/min and pulse rate increases by 15/min or lung crackles develop):

- Stop the fluids.
- Call for help and plan for handover to an advanced provider.

If there is no improvement after the first infusion:

- Call for help. Plan for handover to an advanced provider at a centre with blood transfusion capabilities.
- Give fluid at 4 ml per kilogram over 1 hour while awaiting transfer to the advanced provider.

If the child displays signs of improvement (improved capillary refill, lower pulse rate and respiratory rate):

- Switch to oral or nasogastric rehydration with ReSoMal (low sodium oral rehydration solution) 10 ml per kilogram per hour for up to 10 hours.
- Transfer to a malnutrition unit.

SPECIAL CONSIDERATIONS:

Children with severe anaemia and poor perfusion need urgent handover to an advanced provider and unit with the capacity for blood transfusion.

Children who need IV fluids, but in whom bolus fluids are not indicated should be given maintenance fluids.

See the WHO Child Health publications page (www.who.int/maternal_child_adolescent/documents/child/) for recommended maintenance fluid rates in children.

Circulation skill station assessments

Skills station marking criteria	1st pass	2nd pass	3rd pass
Safety: Personal protective equipment used or states intent to use			
Skill 1 – Assess circulation			
Look for anxiety, confusion, AMS			
Feel for pulse: rate, quality			
Assess capillary refill: >3 seconds indicates poor perfusion			
Assess skin colour and temperature			
Verbalize to measure other vital signs: respiratory rate and blood pressure			
Comments:			

INTRO
ABCDE
TRAUMA
BREATHING
SHOCK
AMS
SKILLS
GLOSSARY
REFS & QUICK CARDS

Skill 2 – Bleeding control: direct pressure

Put on gloves

Uses gauze or another clean, non-adherent dressing, apply firm pressure to the wound

Verbalize to not use bulky dressings

Apply firm pressure as directly as possible to the source of bleeding, usually with two or three fingers

Demonstrate how to elevate a limb with a wound above the heart

Verbalize to not remove the first dressing

Apply second dressing with firm pressure when wound continues to bleed

Apply bandage when bleeding ceased

Verbalize the need to call for help

Comments:

Skill 3 – Bleeding control: deep wound packing

Put on gloves

Identify deep or gaping wound as an indication for deep wound packing

Assesses pulses, capillary refill and sensation after dressing or splinting any wound

Irrigate with 1L clean water before packing.

Use gauze or another clean, compact material to pack the space within the wound

Put additional gauze on top of the wound surface and apply direct pressure with your gloved hand or a bandage wrapped firmly around the wound/limb

If a wound is on a limb and requires packing, consider applying a splint to reduce the risk of re-bleeding

Assesses pulses, capillary refill and sensation after dressing or splinting any wound

State that a deep wound pack should not be left in place for more than 24 hours because of the risk of infection

Comments:

Skill 4 – Bleeding control: tourniquet

Identify continued bleeding as an indication for a tourniquet

States intent to use a blood pressure cuff or thick band or piece of cloth or belt (the wider, the better) after padding skin

Identifies appropriate location for tourniquet

States to tighten tourniquet until the distal pulses disappear. Then re-assess the bleeding to see if it has stopped

States to secure tightened tourniquet in place

States plan to release for 10 minutes every 2 hours. Only re-apply if bleeding resumes

States documentation time of tourniquet placement

States will not leave tourniquet on for more than 2 hours without consulting advanced provider

Comments:

Skill 5 – Uterine massage for postpartum haemorrhage

States to call for help and initiate handover/transfer

States the indication for performing uterine massage

States the need to prepare oxytocin and IV fluid

States that the goal is to compress the uterus between the hand and bony structures behind the uterus (e.g. sacrum/lower back)

Demonstrates how to cup the uterus through the abdominal wall to ensure that it stays under the hand

Demonstrates how to apply strong pressure toward the patient's back while massaging with a circular motion

States that massaging should not stop until the uterus is contracted (feels hard)

States that the uterus should not become relaxed (soft) after uterine massage has stopped. If it does, resume uterine massage

States to continuously re-asses for vaginal bleeding and perform frequent vital signs

Comments:

Skill 6 – Inserting an iv cannula

Prepare equipment: gloves, IV cannula, administration set , fluids, IV tourniquet, swab

Tell the patient what you are about to do

Place IV tourniquet on limb

Identify a straight vein

Clean the skin over the vein

Remove the safety covering and insert the cannula, keeping cannula flat and in line with vein

When flashback is achieved, advance needle slightly and then slide cannula over needle into the vein

Hold this in place and withdraw the needle while putting pressure over base of cannula

Remove the IV tourniquet

Flush with saline or connect IV line

INTRO

ABCDE

TRAUMA

BREATHING

SHOCK

AMS

SKILLS

GLOSSARY

REFS & QUICK CARDS

Secure with tape or dressing
States to check IV site daily to assess for redness or signs of infection
Disposes of any sharps appropriately
Comments:

Skill 7 – Recognizing conditions requiring IV fluid re-adjustment

State the special considerations for fluid resuscitation: malnutrition/severe anaemia/fluid overload
State how to assess for fluid overload: difficulty in breathing with crackles on chest exam, lower body swelling (usually in the legs), unable to lie flat due to shortness of breath, distended neck veins
State ways to adjust fluids in patients in shock with fluid overload: • Small amounts of fluids (250–500 ml boluses in adults) • Slow the rate of fluids • Monitor closely for signs of worsening fluid overload
Verbalize how to assess for signs of severe anaemia
State ways to adjust fluids in patients with severe anaemia: • Slow the rate of fluids • Monitor closely for signs of fluid overload
State need for rapid handover/transfer to a centre capable of blood transfusion
Verbalize how to assess muscle wasting in severe malnutrition
Demonstrate how to assess for bilateral oedema in the feet
State ways to adjust fluids in patients with severe malnutrition: • Give oral fluids if possible • Add dextrose to IV fluids or give dextrose with IV fluids • Slow the rate of fluids • Monitor closely for signs of fluid overload
Comments:

Skill 8 – IV fluid resuscitation for shock

Verbalize caution in administering IV fluid in a malnourished, anaemic or fluid-overloaded patient
Insert an IV cannula as described above
Attach the IV cannula to the correct fluid for administration
Fluid administration for an adult should be normal saline or Ringer's Lactate
States fluid administration for shock in an adult should be 1L given over <30 minutes

Assess perfusion, if still in shock, give another 1L bolus over <30 minutes

State that, if still in shock after 2 L IV fluids, suspect ongoing blood loss and plan for handover to higher-level care

Give mechanism for modifying fluid for an adult if severe malnutrition, severe anaemia or fluid overload is present: give fluid in smaller boluses and re-assess frequently for signs of worsening fluid overload

Signs of fluid overload are:

Fluid in the lungs and difficulty in breathing

- Oedema
- Patient is unable to lie flat
- Distended neck veins

For a child in shock (WITHOUT severe malnutrition, anaemia or overload):

- Obtain the child's weight
- Give 10–20 ml/kg normal saline or Lactated Ringer's over 30 minutes
- Re-assess after the bolus, if no improvement, repeat bolus
- If shock persists, transfer

For a child in shock (WITH severe malnutrition, anaemia or overload):

- Weigh the child
- State that these children need specialized IV fluids
  - Ringer's Lactate with 5% glucose
  - Half-strength Darrow's solution with 5% glucose
  - 0.45% (HALF) normal saline with 5% glucose
- Give 10–15ml/kg IV fluid over 1 hour
- Re-assess the child every 5–10 minutes while receiving fluids
- State if no improvement, transfer

Verbalize to stop IV fluid in any patient if signs of fluid overload develop

Dispose of any sharps appropriately

Comments:

Competency demonstrated	YES	NO
Remediation required	YES	NO
Signature of Facilitator:		

4. EXTENDED PHYSICAL EXAMINATION SKILL STATIONS

EXTENDED PHYSICAL EXAMINATION SKILL STATION: NEUROLOGIC EXAM

Glasgow Coma Scale (GCS)

The GCS is a 15-point scale for assessing and monitoring people with head injury. The person is assessed for eye opening, verbal and motor response, and given a score for the highest level of function in each area. The totals are combined to determine the overall score. The lower the score, the more severe the head injury may be. Please note that the lowest score a patient can receive is 3.

Severe head injury – GCS 8 or less

Moderate head injury – GCS 9–12

Mild head injury – GCS 13–15

Calculating The Glasgow Coma Score (GCS)

Glasgow Coma Score (GCS)		
Function	**Response**	**Score**
Eyes (4)	Open spontaneously	4
	Open to command	3
	Open to pain	2
	None	1
Verbal (5)	Normal	5
	Confused talk	4
	Inappropriate words	3
	Inappropriate sounds	2
	None	1
Motor (6)	Obeys command	6
	Localizes pain	5
	Flexes limbs normally to pain	4
	Flexes limbs abnormally to pain	3
	Extends limbs to pain	2
	None	1

AVPU Scale

The AVPU scale is a simplified assessment that can give you an indication of level of consciousness by assessing response to stimuli. The AVPU scale is particularly useful for children and infants.

- **A= Alert.** People who are fully awake and interactive (even if not fully oriented) are alert.
- **V= Voice.** Those who are not fully alert before stimulus (may have eyes closed or appear sleepy), but do respond to voice without being touched (the response may be words, moaning or movement).
- **P= Pain.** Those who do not respond to voice, but do respond to pain: hard chest (sternal) rub in adults, pinch to the sole of the foot in children, or pinch to bridge of nose in suspected spinal injury. The response may be words, moaning or movement.
- **U= Unresponsive.** Those who do not make any movement or verbal response to painful stimuli are unresponsive.
- For any patient who is P or U on the AVPU scale, stop and return to the ABCDE as rapid intervention may be needed to protect the airway.

INTRO

ABCDE

TRAUMA

BREATHING

SHOCK

AMS

SKILLS

GLOSSARY

REFS & QUICK CARDS

EXTENDED PHYSICAL EXAM SKILL STATION: SECONDARY SURVEY TRAUMA ASSESSMENT

A secondary survey (head-to-toe assessment) of an injured person is conducted ONLY when the ABCDE has been completed and life-threatening complications have been addressed. The purpose of a head-to-toe assessment is to identify all injuries, plan ongoing management and plan the appropriate disposition. If the person deteriorates during the head-to-toe assessment, stop and re-assess the ABCDE immediately. Ensure clothes have been removed but the person is kept warm with gown, sheet or blanket.

For this session use the workbook section on secondary survey from the TRAUMA module.

Extended physical examination skill station assessment

Skills station marking criteria	1st pass	2nd pass	3rd pass
Safety: Personal protective equipment used or verbalized use			
HEAD-TO-TOE TRAUMA ASSESSMENT			
Skill 1 – HEENT examination			
Look at scalp, face, eyes, and in mouth, nose, ears			
Listen for stridor, gurgling or other airway sounds			
Feel for abnormal facial bone or jaw movement, loose teeth, or crepitus.			
Comments:			
Skill 2 – Neck examination			
Look for neck wounds, trauma, haematoma or distended neck veins			
Feel for air in tissue or pain/deformity of the cervical spine			
Check for reduced ability to move neck or pain			
Comments:			
Skill 3 – Chest examination			
Look for bruising, uneven chest movement, burns			
Listen for breath sounds, muffled heart sounds			
Feel for crepitus			
Comments:			
Skill 4 – Abdominal examination			
Look for distension, wounds, bruising, burns			
Feel for rebound tenderness, guarding, location of pain			
Comments:			

Skill 5 – Pelvis and genitourinary examination

Look for bruising, lacerations, blood, priapism, urine colour

Feel for pelvis instability or tenderness

Comments:

Skill 6 – Extremity examination

Look for swelling, bruising, deformity or open fractures, wounds, pale extremity

Feel for pulses, cold extremity, tenderness, firm/painful muscle compartments

Comments:

Skill 7 – spine/back examination

Log roll patient with assistance

Look for bruising or deformity

Feel for tenderness, deformity in spine and scapulae

Comments:

Skill 8 – Skin examination

Look for bruising, abrasions, lacerations, burns

Comments:

Skill 9 – Neurologic examination

Check level of consciousness (AVPU or GCS)

Check movement and strength in each limb

Check for priapism

Check sensation on face, chest, limbs

Comments:

Competency demonstrated	YES	NO
Remediation required	YES	NO
Facilitator's signature:		

5. IMMOBILIZATION SKILL STATIONS

Approach to spinal immobilization

There are two types of spinal immobilization: cervical spine and thoracic/lumbar spine. Together, these are called full spine immobilization. Immobilization stabilizes the bones to avoid further injury to the spine. **Provide spinal immobilization to any person with a history of polytrauma who is unconscious; or who is conscious and has neck pain, spine tenderness, numbness or weakness.** Remember, immobilized patients cannot move normally and are at a higher risk of airway blockage (by secretions or vomit) and pressure sore development. Monitor closely.

IMMOBILIZATION SKILL STATION: CERVICAL SPINE IMMOBILIZATION

To immobilize the cervical spine:

- Keep the patient flat on his or her back and face up on a level surface such as a bed.
- Tell the patient what you are doing.
- Hold the patient's head in line with the spine with two hands on either side of the head.
- Prevent the patient's neck from moving with locally available materials (towel rolls, newspaper, sandbags, or bags of IV fluids) or cervical collar if available. These can be secured to the head with tape (plaster) but should never be secured to the bed. (If the patient vomits, you will not be able to turn him or her and if the patient falls, the tape (plaster) could cause a cervical spine injury.)
- If the patient vomits, use the log-roll technique (see below) to turn the whole patient onto his or her side, keeping the head in line with the body.
- Keep someone with the patient at all times to watch the airway.
- Remember, a patient who has severe pain/injury elsewhere may not be able to feel neck pain, even if there is a fracture. A concerning mechanism should raise suspicion.

INTRO

ABCDE

TRAUMA

BREATHING

SHOCK

AMS

SKILLS

GLOSSARY

REFS & QUICK CARDS

IMMOBILIZATION SKILL STATION: LOG ROLL

To move any immobilized patient or anyone with a suspected spine injury (e.g. if the patient has to vomit or needs to be transferred), use the log-roll technique (see figure):

- Ask for assistance. Ideally, have one person at the head to hold the neck, one or two people to hold the body and one for the legs.
- The provider at the head must keep the head, neck and torso aligned with the rest of the spine. The provider should place their forearms tightly alongside the head with hands gripping the shoulders to keep the head and neck in line with the rest of the spine. Keep this alignment when turning the patient.
- The person controlling the head and neck leads the team and will say, "1–2-3 roll" to guide timing of the roll for all assistants.
- Working together, roll the patient onto his or her side, keeping the spine in line.
- During the roll, the person providing head and neck control must ensure the cervical spine remains aligned with the rest of the spine. The people rolling the body should also ensure that the rest of the spine stays in as straight a line as possible.
- When the patient is turned onto one side, a provider can examine the back, place or remove a backboard and/or manage back wounds as needed.
- To lie the patient flat again, the person controlling the head and neck uses the "1–2–3 roll" command to ensure coordinated movement.
- Always remove a backboard as soon as possible using the log-roll technique. Time on a backboard increases the risk of pressure sores. Check pressure areas frequently using the log roll.

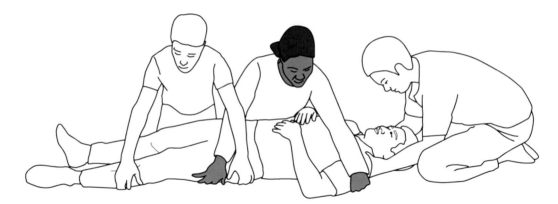

Preparing for log roll

IMMOBILIZATION SKILL STATION: FULL SPINAL IMMOBILIZATION

To immobilize the thoracic and lumbar spine (see previous section for cervical spine immobilization):

- Immobilize the cervical spine as in previous section.
- Keep the person on a flat surface with instructions to lie flat and not to move.
- For transport, log roll the patient onto a flat surface (such as a backboard) to prevent movement of the spine. Do not attach the backboard to the bed, as you will be unable to log roll (see above) if needed.
- Before immobilizing, be sure there is no glass or debris on or under the patient's back. Use the log roll to check. Immobilized patients must be checked regularly to avoid pressure point wounds.
- If the person needs to vomit, use the log-roll technique to roll the person to the side so that no vomit enters the airway.
- Spine boards should ONLY be used to move patients. Leaving patients on spine boards for long periods of time can cause pressure sores. Remove patients from boards as soon as they arrive at the facility and can be laid flat.

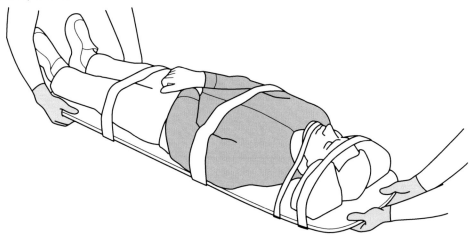

Spinal immobilization for moving a patient

IMMOBILIZATION SKILL STATION: POSITIONING OF THE PREGNANT PATIENT

- If a patient is over 20 weeks pregnant and needs spinal immobilization, immobilize the spine as above. Then place padding under the side of the board near the back and hips to tilt the patient onto her left side. This helps to prevent compression of the large internal blood vessels by the pregnant uterus which could decrease blood returning to the heart.

INTRO

ABCDE

TRAUMA

BREATHING

SHOCK

AMS

SKILLS

GLOSSARY

REFS & QUICK CARDS

IMMOBILIZATION SKILL STATION: RECOVERY POSITION

- If the patient is unconscious or semiconscious and if there is NO TRAUMA, place the patient on his or her left side. Stabilize the patient by bending the top leg forward. The left arm should be straight with the patient's head resting on the arm to elevate the head and position the mouth downward. This position will allow for vomit and other secretions to drain from the mouth with less risk of airway obstruction. This is called the recovery position (see figure).

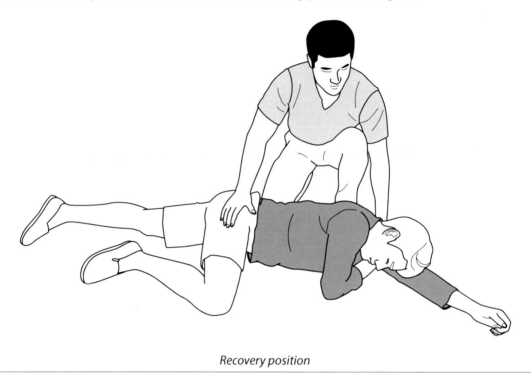

Recovery position

IMMOBILIZATION SKILL STATION: FRACTURE IMMOBILIZATION

FRACTURE IMMOBILIZATION

Splints are used for immobilizing suspected fractured limbs, preventing pain caused by movement of broken bones and minimizing further bleeding and damage. Always assess and record perfusion of the limb beyond the fracture by assessing pulses and capillary refill time. Always assess pulses, capillary refill and sensation **before AND after** dressing or splinting any wound.

- If no perfusion (limb cold, pale, no pulse, slow or no capillary refill), rapid re-alignment (reduction) of the limb is required to restore circulation.
- If there is still no perfusion after re-alignment of the limb, splint and plan for rapid handover/ transfer to a specialist unit.
- If you cannot re-align the limb, rapidly handover/transfer to an advanced provider.

Goal of fracture management:

- Restore circulation
- Treat and reduce pain
- Prevent further injury and bleeding
- Re-align bony fragments so that healing and union can take place and normal function is restored

Splinting materials include:

- Padding to protect the skin and allow swelling
- Pre-formed splint for base or modified local resources
- Bandages to secure the splint
- Adhesive tape (plaster)

Before applying a splint, tell the person what you are doing and give pain relief.

- Remove clothing to clearly see the injury.
- Remove all jewelry.

- Check pulses, capillary refill, sensation and movement of the limb. Document this before and after application of the splint.
- Size the splint to immobilize the joint **above** and **below** the fracture site.
- If the limb is visibly deformed and pulses beyond the fracture are weak or absent, first straighten (reduce) the fracture prior to applying the splint. Do not force realignment of a deformed limb if the limb has a good pulse.
- Place the joint in the desired position and if the injury involves fingers or toes, pad between toes and fingers.
- If stocking gauze is available, place it over the limb without wrinkles to avoid skin damage.
- Pad the side of the splint that will be in contact with the skin, and pad the limb, especially bony protrusions (like the elbow).
- Wrap the limb and splint with a bandage to hold the splint. Ask the patient how it feels to ensure it is not too tight. The splint should be secure, but remember that the limb will swell, so it is important that the splint and bandaging are not too tight.
- Check pulses, sensation and movement of the limb following the application of the splint and every hour afterward.

INTRO

ABCDE

TRAUMA

BREATHING

SHOCK

AMS

SKILLS

GLOSSARY

REFS & QUICK CARDS

FRACTURE IMMOBILIZATION: OPEN

Consider an open fracture if there is a wound near a fracture site. Open fracture sites can often be contaminated and will require cleaning and potentially surgical debridement before the fracture can be fixed. If an open fracture is suspected, plan for handover/transfer to a surgical or orthopaedic unit after splinting.

- Give pain relief prior to splinting.
- Control haemorrhage with direct pressure. In limb amputation, if bleeding is uncontrolled apply tourniquet (see above), commence fluid resuscitation and plan for rapid handover/transfer.
- Straighten (reduce) the limb if there are signs of poor perfusion or absent pulses in the limb.
- Remove any dirt, grass, obvious glass or other debris from the wound and irrigate the wound with 2 litres of normal saline.
- Cover the wound with saline-soaked gauze.
- Splint as above, but leave a window so you can continue to monitor the wound.
- In amputation, cover wound with sterile, saline-soaked gauze or towel.
- Give tetanus vaccination.
- Begin IV antibiotics.

IMMOBILIZATION SKILL STATION: APPLYING A PELVIC BINDER

Pelvic fractures can cause life-threatening haemorrhage by damaging blood vessels adjacent to the fractures. If a person has been injured and has pain in and around the pelvis, apply a binder (see figures). As the pelvis is shaped in a ring, the binder will bring together the displaced bones and help limit internal bleeding. Signs of pelvic fractures include pain or abnormal movement of the pelvis on exam; bruising around the hips, at the top of legs, or to the genitals; and signs and symptoms of shock.

- Place bed sheet or similar under the pelvis. If the bed sheet is wide, fold it over so that it spans from the lower back to the end of the buttocks.
- You may need to log roll the patient in order to get the binder in position.
- The sheet should be centered over the greater trochanters (hip bones, as demonstrated by the instructor) and firmly cross-over at the front.
- Pull firmly and tie, but do not cause the person undue pain. It should feel firm but not overly painful.
- Document what time the pelvic binder was applied.
- Check the binder each hour. Confirm that the binder is still applying pressure around the pelvis. Ensure that that skin is intact where the binder has been applied and around the genitals.

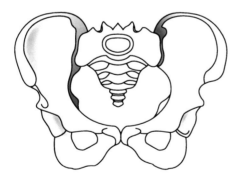

Normal pelvis

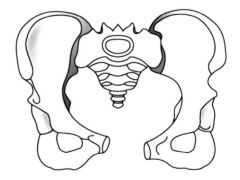

Open pelvic fracture

Pelvic immobilization

Immobilization skill station assessments

Skills station marking criteria	1st pass	2nd pass	3rd pass
Safety: Personal protective equipment used or verbalized use			
Skill 1 – Cervical spinal immobilization			
Keep the patient lying flat.			
Tell the patient what you are doing.			
Hold the patient's head in line with the spine using your two hands on either side of the head.			
A partner should use rolled sheets, shoes, or IV fluid bags on either side of the head. May be secured with tape (plaster) but do not secure to the bed.			
State that if the patient vomits, log-roll technique will be used to protect the airway, keeping the head aligned with the rest of the body.			
Comments:			
Skill 2 – Log roll			
State indications for a log roll.			
Ask for assistance.			
Place one person at the head to hold the neck, one or two people to hold the body and one for the legs.			
The person with head control must hold the cervical spine firmly aligned with the rest of the spine before and during the roll.			
When the provider at the head and neck instructs, roll the patient onto the side. Use "1–2–3 roll" to guide the roll.			
The person controlling the head and neck uses the "1–2–3 roll" to return the patient to his or her back.			

INTRO

ABCDE

TRAUMA

BREATHING

SHOCK

AMS

SKILLS

GLOSSARY

REFS & QUICK CARDS

State that the patient should be removed from the backboard as soon as possible to prevent pressure sores.

Comments:

Skill 3 – Full spine immobilization

State indication for full spine immobilization.

Ask for assistance to help with the movement.

Perform log roll on to backboard for transfer.

Ensure no glass or debris on or under the patient's back.

Secure patient to backboard device for transfer (Do NOT attach backboard or patient to bed).

State to log roll if patient needs to vomit.

Skill 4 – Positioning of the pregnant patient

Verbalize the indications for positioning (greater than 20 weeks pregnant and needs spinal immobilization).

Left lateral position with cervical spine immobilization and a pillow or wedge under the backboard or bed.

Comments:

Skill 5 – Recovery position

Verbalize the indications.

Controlled manoeuver into left lateral position ensuring open airway.

Appropriately position the patient (top leg bent forward, left arm straight with the patient's head resting on the arm to elevate the head and position the mouth downward).

Comments:

Skill 6 – Fracture immobilization

Remove clothing to clearly see the injury, remove all jewelry.

Check pulses, sensation and movement of the limb and document findings.

Size the splint against the limb. Immobilize the joint above and below the injury.

Identify special considerations:

• Straighten the limb if signs of poor perfusion or absent pulses in the limb.
• Control haemorrhage as needed.
• Remove debris and irrigate an open fracture wound with 2 L of normal saline.
• Cover open fractures with sterile saline gauze.

Place the joint in the desired position.

Pad in between toes and fingers if injury involves digits.

If stockinette is available, place it over the limb without wrinkles or pad the side of the splint that will be in contact with the skin.

Pad the patient's limb, especially bony prominences.

Wrap the limb and splint with a bandage to hold the splint.

Check pulses, sensation and movement of the limb following the application of the splint.

State patients with an open fracture will require tetanus vaccination, if not up to date, and antibiotics.

Comments:

Skill 7 – Applying a pelvic binder

Identify pelvic pain after trauma.

Place bed sheet under the pelvis. If bed sheet is wide, fold it over so that it is the size of the pelvis (lower back to end of buttocks).

Push the binder under the small of the back and pull it into position or log roll patient onto binder.

Centre over the great trochanters (hip bones) and firmly cross over at the front.

Pull firmly and tie, but do not cause the person undue pain. It should feel firm but not overly painful.

Document the time the pelvic binder was applied.

Comments:

Competency demonstrated	YES	NO
Remediation required	YES	NO
Signature of facilitator:		

6. WOUND MANAGEMENT SKILL STATIONS

WOUND MANAGEMENT: GENERAL WOUND MANAGEMENT

- Haemorrhage control: stop bleeding as above.
- Prevent infection:
  - Clean wound of blood clots, dirt, dead or dying tissue, foreign bodies.
  - Clean skin around the wound thoroughly with soap and water or antiseptic.
  - Thoroughly wash out wound by flushing with at least 1 litre of clean water.
    - The water should be under pressure to thoroughly clean the wound. To create a high pressure stream, use a syringe (with 14 g needle or IV catheter attached) or poke a small hole in a clean bottle and squeeze the bottle.
    - Be sure to use the entire litre.
  - If not vaccinated or not up to date, give tetanus vaccination.

- Dressing wounds:
  - Dress wound with sterile gauze if available.
  - Use a pressure dressing if the wound is still bleeding.
  - Check perfusion (capillary refill and/or distal pulses) and sensation beyond the wound before AND after dressing wounds.

- Pain management:
  - Give local anaesthetic before cleaning the wound if staff and equipment are available.
  - Splint large lacerations and fractures.

WOUND MANAGEMENT: BURN MANAGEMENT

It is important to cover burns early in order to keep the area moist and reduce the risk of infection. Burns can be very painful so ensure you give pain relief.

- Use sterile technique and normal saline to clean the burn.
- Carefully remove any loose, dead skin and broken, tense or infected blisters.

- Apply a non-adherent dressing to the burn to provide a moist healing environment. Clean clear plastic wrap can be used over the burn as an interim measure and if you are transferring the person to a surgical unit shortly.
- Ensure the entire burn is covered with the dressing.
- If the person has presented with an old burn that is now infected, apply a topical antibiotic (such as bacitracin or silver sulfadiazine). This person may also require IV or intramuscular antibiotics.
- If there is delay in handover or transfer, ensure the dressings are changed daily. Always give pain control with dressing changes.

ADULT BURN MANAGEMENT: DETERMINE TOTAL BODY SURFACE AREA (TBSA)

This is used to calculate the fluids needed using the Parkland Formula. Use the Rule of Nines body chart for adults and modified chart for children and infants (see figure).

The body is divided into portions that each make up 9% of the total body surface. Children have different percentages due to the different body proportions, such as a larger head and smaller limbs (see figures).

- Assess the person using the diagram below.
- Note the areas of burn and shade them in on the diagram.
- Next to where you are shading, write the burn depth (see burn depth estimate below).
- Once you have marked the diagram (front and back) with all the burns you have assessed on the person, add the percentages.
- This will give you the total burn surface area (TBSA).

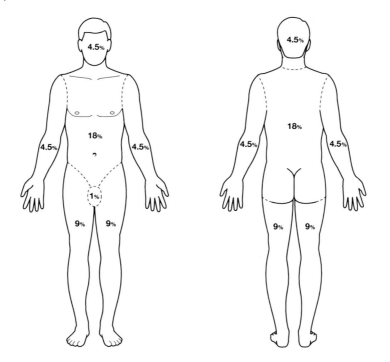

Burn surface area in adults

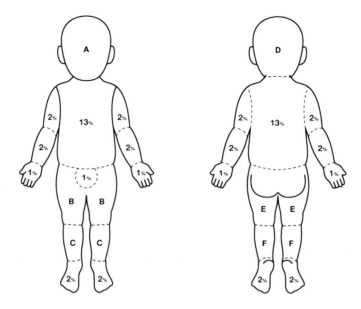

Burn surface area in children

PAEDIATRIC BURN MANAGEMENT: DETERMINE TOTAL BODY SURFACE AREA (TBSA)

Area	By age in years			
	0	1	5	10
Head (A or D)	10%	9%	7%	6%
Thigh (B or E)	3%	3%	4%	5%
Leg (C or F)	2%	3%	3%	3%

BURN MANAGEMENT: ESTIMATE DEPTH OF BURN

The best way to estimate burn depth is by gently pressing two fingers onto the burn to assess capillary refill.

• Put gloves on.

• With care, press down on the centre of the burn with two fingertips for 3–4 seconds, and then let go. The faster the capillary refill the more superficial the burn is.

• Now assess the outer edge of the burn (burn depth can vary for different areas of the burn).

• Use the chart below to guide your assessment findings.

Burn type	Skin findings
Superficial (formerly first degree)	• Red or pink • Painful, skin intact, no blisters • When pressed, skin is pink with quick capillary refill
Partial thickness (formerly second degree)	• Red or mottled red • Intact or broken blisters, wet • Painful • May temporarily turn white when pressed then red colour returns
Full thickness (formerly third degree)	• White or black • Leathery and dry • No sensation • When pressed, no change in colour

BURN MANAGEMENT: FLUID RESUSCITATION IN BURN INJURY

As discussed in the TRAUMA module, an adult or child with a burn injury may require fluid resuscitation. Start fluid resuscitation in the following cases:

• Full or partial thickness burns greater than or equal to 15% total burn surface area in adults.
• Full or partial thickness burns greater than or equal to 10% total burn surface area in children.

BURN MANAGEMENT: PARKLAND FORMULA CALCULATION FOR THE FIRST 24 HOURS

> ### 4 ml IV fluid   X   weight in kilograms   X   % total burn surface area*
>
> *% total burn surface area = % partial thickness burn area + % full thickness burn area
>
> (% superficial burn area is NOT used in the calculation)

The **Parkland Formula** is a fluid resuscitation management strategy for the initial 24 hours following a burn. Patients presenting beyond 24 hours after the initial burn will also need fluid resuscitation, but the Parkland Formula is not used beyond 24 hours.

• The first half of the fluid should be given within the first 8 hours after the burn (NOT after arrival to care).
• The second half is to be given over the subsequent 16 hours.
• For adults, give normal saline or Ringer's Lactate.
• For children, use a dextrose-containing fluid (Ringer's Lactate with 5% dextrose or normal saline with 5% dextrose for initial resuscitation). If no dextrose-containing fluids are available, give an additional dose of dextrose (either IV or orally) with IV fluids (see MEDICATIONS).

For ongoing care of children, the Parkland emergency resuscitation fluids calculated above MUST BE ADDED to any required maintenance fluids based on hospital care protocols (see WHO Pocket book of hospital care for children, 2013).

Your facilitator will review examples using the Parkland Formula.

REMEMBER: Patients with serious burns to >15% of their body, burns involving the hand, face, groin area, joints, or burns that go completely around the body or a body part need to be transferred/handed over for specialized care.

WOUND MANAGEMENT: SNAKE BITE BANDAGING AND IMMOBILIZATION

Note: When possible, take a picture of the snake and send with the patient.

Immobilizing a limb after a snake bite is important to reduce movement and absorption of venom.

• Always assess pulses, capillary refill and sensation **before and after** dressing or splinting any wound.

• You may choose to use a broad pressure bandage and wrap upwards from the lower portion of the bite. The bandage should be firm, but should not cut off pulses in the limb. Extend the bandage as high up the limb as possible.

  – This is recommended if the snakes in your area produce a toxin that damages the nerves, causes paralysis, causes the person to become very ill or if there will be prolonged transport time.

  – This is NOT recommended if the snakes in your area produce toxins that primarily cause tissue damage near the wound and do not cause body-wide symptoms.

• Bind a splint to the limb to immobilize as much of the limb as possible.

• Note the time the bandage was placed.

• Keep the person still and lying down.

• DO NOT put a tourniquet around the snake bite or limb.

• DO NOT cut the bite out as this will lead to unnecessary bleeding.

• DO NOT suck on the bite to remove the venom.

Wound management skill station assessments

Skills station marking criteria	1st pass	2nd pass	3rd pass
Safety: Personal protective equipment used or verbalized use			
SKILL 1– General wound management			
Haemorrhage control: stops bleeding as per earlier taught skill.			
Preventing infection			
Cleans wound of blood clots, dirt and foreign bodies.			
Cleans skin around the wound thoroughly with soap and water or antiseptic.			
Thoroughly washes out wound by flushing with water (state 1 litre of clean water or more).			
Gives tetanus vaccination as needed.			
Dressing wounds			
Assesses pulses, capillary refill and sensation before dressing or splinting any wound.			
Dresses wound with sterile gauze if available.			
Applies pressure dressing if the wound is still bleeding.			
Checks perfusion beyond the wound (capillary refill and/or distal pulses) before and after dressing wounds.			
Pain management			

Gives local anaesthetic before cleaning the wound if staff and equipment are available.

Splints large lacerations and fractures.

Assesses pulses, capillary refill and sensation after dressing or splinting any wound.

Comments:

BURN MANAGEMENT

Skill 2 – Burn wound management

Uses a sterile technique and normal saline to clean the burn.

Removes any loose, dead skin and broken, tense or infected blisters.

Applies a non-adherent dressing to the burn to provide a moist healing environment.

Ensures the entire burn is covered with the dressing.

Considers antibiotics.

States transfer or handover plan.

Comments:

Skill 3 – Fluid resuscitation in burn injury

Correctly states indications:
• Partial or full thickness burns greater than or equal to 15% total burn surface area in adult.
• Partial or full thickness burns greater than or equal to 10% total burn surface area in children.

Estimates depth of burn.

Determines total body surface area (TBSA).

Calculates Parkland Formula.

Explains delivery of fluids.

(First half in first 8 hrs; second half in next 16 hrs)

Chooses correct fluid for initial bolus.

(Children weighing less than 20 kg: Ringer's Lactate with 5% dextrose, normal saline with 5% dextrose)

Comments:

Skill 4: Snake bite bandaging and immobilization

Uses a broad pressure bandage and wrap upwards from the lower portion of the bite.

Extends the bandage as high up the limb as possible.

Immobilize as much of the limb as possible with a splint.		
Notes the time the bandage went on.		
Keeps the person still.		
States DO NOT put a tourniquet around the snake bite or limb.		
States DO NOT cut or suck on the bite wound.		
Comments:		

Competency demonstrated	YES	NO
Remediation required	YES	NO
Facilitator's signature:		

7. Medication administration skill discussion

The table below summarizes the medications discussed in this course, which represent only a very basic set of treatments for emergency conditions. They have been included based on their wide availability, their appropriateness for use by all of the frontline providers targeted by this course, their feasibility of use in pre-hospital or facility settings, and for their potential importance as early treatments for emergency conditions. Be sure to check locally available drug concentrations, as these can vary. The most common concentrations are used in this table for dosing reference. Almost every condition discussed will require additional treatments beyond these, and many important emergency treatments that may be used by advanced providers are not included here.

Table: Medications used in the Basic Emergency Care course

Drug indication	Dosage	Adverse effects
Adrenaline (Epinephrine) Anaphylaxis/severe allergic reaction and severe wheezing [see ABCDE, DIB]	**Solution: 1 mg in 1 ml ampoule (1:1000)** **Note:** • **The doses below are for intramuscular not IV administration.** • **The preferred site for injection is the outer mid-thigh.** **Adults:** **Intramuscular(IM):** 50 kg or above: 0.5 mg **IM** (0.5 ml of 1:1000) 40 kg: 0.4 mg **IM** (0.4 ml of 1:1000) 30 kg: 0.3 mg **IM** (0.3 ml of 1:1000) • May repeat at 5-minute intervals **Paediatrics:** **Anaphylaxis**: 0.15 mg **IM** (0.15 ml of 1:1000), repeat every 5–15 minutes as needed **Severe asthma**: 0.01 mg/kg **IM** up to 0.3 mg, repeat every 15 minutes as needed	• Anxiety/fear • Palpitations • Tachycardia (elevated heart rate) • Dizziness • Sweating • Nausea • Vomiting • Hyperglycaemia (elevated blood glucose) • Chest pain • High blood pressure • Tissue necrosis at injection site

Drug indication	Dosage	Adverse effects
Antibiotics	Specific drugs in this category will be determined by local treatment protocols and availability. These should include a broad-spectrum regimen for life-threatening infections that can be used empirically (before the infectious source is definitively identified) in very ill patients.	• Allergic reactions • Gastrointestinal upset • Other specific effects vary by antibiotic
Acetylsalicylic acid (Aspirin) Suspected heart attack	**Tablet: 100 mg, 300 mg** **Oral:** 300 mg (preferably chewed or dispersed in water) given immediately as a single dose. Do NOT give aspirin until evaluated by an advanced provider if there is: 1. any active bleeding, or 2. chest pain that is sudden, maximum at onset, sharp and tearing, and radiating to the back (can indicate a tear in the aorta).	• Gastrointestinal irritation with blood loss • Tinnitus • Anaphylaxis
Benzodiazepines – Diazepam Seizures/convulsions [see AMS]	**Tablet: 2 mg, 5 mg** **Solution: 5 mg/1 ml ampoule** **Adults:** First dose: 10 mg slow IV push OR 20 mg rectally Second dose after 10 minutes: 5 mg slow IV push or 10 mg rectally Maximum IV dose: 30 mg **Children:** First dose: 0.2 mg/kg slow IV push or 0.5 mg/kg rectally. Can repeat half of first dose after 10 minutes if seizures/convulsions continue. Maximum IV dose: 20 mg **Do not give second dose if respiratory rate is less than 10 breaths per minute.** **Do not give diazepam intramuscularly (unpredictable absorption).** **How to give rectal diazepam:** • Draw up the dose from an ampoule of diazepam into a small syringe (tuberculin if available). Base the dose on the weight of the child, when possible. • Remove the needle. • Insert the syringe 4–5 cm into the rectum, and inject the diazepam solution. • Hold the buttocks together for a few minutes.	• Sedation • Respiratory depression • Low blood pressure • Bradycardia (low heart rate) • Nausea and vomiting • Abdominal cramps

INTRO

ABCDE

TRAUMA

BREATHING

SHOCK

AMS

SKILLS

GLOSSARY

REFS & QUICK CARDS

Drug indication	Dosage	Adverse effects
Glucose (dextrose) Hypoglycaemia (low blood sugar) [see ABCDE, ALTERED MENTAL STATUS]	**Solution: 50% dextrose (D50), 25% dextrose (D25), 10% dextrose (D10)** **NOTE: Dextrose should NEVER be given intramuscularly as it may cause serious tissue damage.** **Adults and children greater than 40 kg:** 25–50 ml **IV** of D50, or 125–250 ml **IV** of D10 **Children up to 40 kg:** 5 ml/kg **IV** 10% dextrose (D10) D10 is preferred in children under 40 kg. If D10 is not available, you can use the Rule of 50 to remember the equivalent amount of dextrose in another solution. All of the following contain the same amount of dextrose: 5 ml of D10 2 ml of D25 1 ml of D50 **If no IV access:** Place 2–5 ml of 50% dextrose in buccal space (inside the cheek) **OR** Give sugar solution (1 level teaspoon of sugar moistened with water every 10–20 minutes) in buccal space	• Hyperglycaemia (high blood glucose) • Dizziness • Skin necrosis if injected outside the vein

Drug indication	Dosage	Adverse effects
Magnesium sulphate Eclampsia or pregnant with seizure/convulsion [see ALTERED MENTAL STATUS]	**Solution forms:** **1 g in 2 ml ampoule (50%)** **5 g in 10 ml ampoule (50%)** **To give IV, make a 20% solution:** *add 3 ml of sterile saline to the 2 ml ampule **OR** *add 15 ml of sterile saline to the 10 ml ampoule. **Loading dose (IV + IM):** * **4 g IV** (dilute to a 20% solution and give 20 ml *slowly* over 20 minutes) **AND** *10 g IM (intramuscular): 5 g (10 ml of 50% solution) with 1 ml of 2% lidocaine **in** upper outer quadrant of **each** buttock. Magnesium can cause low blood pressure; monitor carefully. **IF unable to give IV, give 10 g IM injection only (as above, 5 g in each buttock).** **If seizures/convulsions recur:** after 15 minutes give an additional 2 g (10 ml of 20%) IV over 20 minutes. **If transport delayed, continue treatment:** Give 5 g of 50% solution IM with 1 ml of 2% lidocaine every four hours in alternate buttocks.	• Low blood pressure • Respiratory depression • Drowsiness • Confusion • Loss of reflexes • Muscle weakness • Nausea • Vomiting • Flushed skin • Thirst **STOP if:** • Respiratory depression (respiratory rate <16) develops. **Toxicity:** • Low blood pressure • Respiratory depression • Loss of knee jerk • Urine output <100 ml/4 hours
Naloxone Opioid overdose [see ABCDE, ALTERED MENTAL STATUS, DIFFICULTY IN BREATHING]	**Solution: 400 mcg/ml (hydrochloride) in 1 ml ampoule** **IV:** 100 mcg single dose **OR** **IM:** 400 mcg in single dose May repeat every 5 minutes as needed. May require continuous infusion at 0.4 mg/hour for several hours for long-acting opioids.	• Hypertension (high blood pressure) • Cardiac arrhythmias • Hyperventilation • Difficulty in breathing • Agitation *** Naloxone effects only last 1–3 hours. Many opioid medications are longer-acting and may need more doses of naloxone or a naloxone infusion. Any patient treated with naloxone must be monitored closely***

Drug indication	Dosage	Adverse effects
Oxytocin Treatment of postpartum haemorrhage	**Solution: 10 IU in 1 ml ampule** **Initial dose:** Give 10 IU IM **AND** start IV fluids with 20 IU/L at 60 drops/minute. **Once the placenta is delivered, continue** IV fluids with 20 IU/L at 30 drops/minute if still bleeding. **If placenta has to be manually removed or uterus does not contract:** Repeat 10 IU IM. **Continue** IV fluids with 20 IU/L at 20 drops/minute for 1 hour after bleeding stops. **Max Dose:** 3 L of IV fluids containing oxytocin.	• Nausea/vomiting • Headache • Rash • Anaphylaxis • Uterine spasm (at low doses) • Uterine hyperstimulation (at high doses)
Paracetamol (acetaminophen) Mild to moderate pain, fever and headache	**Tablet: 250 mg, 500 mg** **Rectal suppositories: 250 mg, 500 mg** **Adults:** 500mg – 1 g every 6 hours Max 4 g daily or max 2 g daily if liver impairment, cirrhosis **Children:** 10–15 mg/kg up to six times a day	• Rash • Liver damage following overdoses
Salbutamol (albuterol) Severe wheezing [see ABCDE, DIFFICULTY IN BREATHING]	**Where available, can use nebulizer with appropriate dose.** **Inhaler: 100 mcg per puff** **Inhaler with spacer** **Adult:** Prime with five puffs and give two puffs via spacer every two minutes until improved. **Child:** Prime with five puffs and give two puffs into spacer. Keep spacer in the child's mouth for three to five breaths. Repeat until six puffs of the drug have been given to a child < 5 years or 12 puffs for > 5 years of age. Repeat regularly until condition improves. In severe cases, 6 or 12 puffs can be given several times in an hour. Remember: child must be able to seal mouth around spacer opening. Babies will likely require spacer mask or nebulizer. **Nebulizer:** (ADULT) 5mg in 5 ml sterile saline. (CHILD) 2.5mg in 3 ml sterile saline. *For severe wheezing, above doses can be given several times in an hour.*	• Palpitations • Fine tremor • Headache • Tachycardia (high heart rate)
Tetanus vaccination	**Solution: 5 units per 0.5 ml** **IM 0.5 ml** **Give to all injured children whose vaccinations are not up to date and in all adults who have not had this vaccination in the past 5 years. If immunization status is unknown, give vaccination.**	• Pain to injection site • Allergic reaction • Fever • Nausea

8. Transfer and handover skills discussion

This course is intended for providers working in the field, on ambulances and in health-care facilities. Transferring patients from the scene to first facility, or between facilities, require special attention to destination planning, ongoing management and handover.

DESTINATION PLANNING

Many patients treated on the scene will require transport to a health-care facility for further management. Additionally, patients already at a facility may require transfer to a different facility for more advanced care. For example, a pregnant woman with seizures will need handover for advanced care and emergency delivery; a patient with severe burns will require transfer for advanced airway management and surgical care; a patient in shock from blood loss will require handover to a centre capable of blood transfusion.

When planning any transport, make sure that: the level of services at the destination facility matches the needs of the patient (e.g. there is an operating theatre if surgery is needed); that the expected resources are currently available (e.g., the operating theatre is running, and there is blood for transfusion); and that the destination can be reached in the necessary time frame given the patient's condition. Do not delay transport for tests or interventions that are not critical to patient safety if they can be performed at the receiving facility.

Follow local transfer and destination protocols where they exist. Where there are no clear protocols, balance transport times with facility capabilities – the goal is to reach needed care as soon as possible. It is usually better to have a longer initial transport time than to arrange a second transfer because appropriate care was not available at the first destination.

Once the appropriate facility has been determined, communication with a provider at the receiving facility is essential (see 'Handover' below). This will allow the receiving centre to prepare for the patient's arrival and arrange resources (e.g. blood, operating theatre preparation). Follow specific local communication protocols where they exist.

Wherever possible, formal protocols for both pre-hospital transport and transfer between facilities should be in place. These should include explicit criteria for when a patient should be transferred.

TRANSPORT

Transfer includes two aspects: transporting the patient and caring for the patient at all times during transport. One person cannot do both jobs. During transport, at least one provider should always be in the same part of the vehicle as the patient to allow for ongoing monitoring, assessment and management. The ABCDE approach should be used to assess and re-assess ALL patients during transportation; vital signs (including AVPU or GCS) should be checked every 15 minutes, and patients should be closely monitored for response to treatments and for signs of worsening.

Remember to plan overall transportation time and route, and check road conditions and weather. This is essential in order to anticipate the patient's needs during transport (e.g. IV fluid and medication needs). Ensure that the patient and family are aware of the transport plan. Allow a family member to accompany children whenever possible.

HANDOVER

Formal handover should be given any time care is transferred to a new provider, including: between providers within a facility, to or from transport providers, or remotely from a sending facility to a receiving facility provider. In addition to a verbal report at the time a patient is handed over to a new provider, written documentation of the clinical condition and treatment should accompany the patient at all times.

You will practise handover summaries throughout the course in the case scenarios. The Situation, Background, Assessment, Recommendations (SBAR) format is a structured way of communicating key information and can be used for all of the handovers mentioned above. SBAR components and examples are:

SITUATION

- Basic patient information (e.g. age, sex).

- Chief complaint (the patient's initial description of the problem, such as difficulty in breathing for 3 days, or arm pain after a fall, etc.).

BACKGROUND

- The 2–4 most important and relevant aspects of the patient's case and/or condition (these may be elements of the history, physical exam, or testing results, depending on the case).

- Include any important ABCDE findings/interventions.

ASSESSMENT

- What you think is wrong with the patient.

- The reason for the handover/transfer.

RECOMMENDATIONS

- Specific things the new provider should prepare for:
  - next steps in the treatment plan;
  - potential worsening of the patient's condition (e.g. need for close airway observation if inhalation burn is suspected);
  - cautions regarding prior therapies or interventions (e.g. time of last adrenaline dose to anticipate return symptoms, need to monitor mental status if sedating medications have been given, need to monitor 3-way dressing for clotting, etc.).

Examples:

Case 1: A 22 year-old man was riding a motorcycle when he crashed into another vehicle at high speed. He was thrown from his motorcycle and was not wearing a helmet. His airway is open; he has normal breath sounds on both sides of his chest; his pulses are strong and around 90 beats per minute; he is only responsive to pain and has a femur fracture with bone visible in an open wound; there are abrasions on his forehead. You have immobilized his spine, started an IV and splinted the fracture. You and your colleague have transported him from the scene of injury and are handing him over to a hospital provider.

Handover summary: *This is a 22-year-old man who was in a motorcycle crash, was not wearing a helmet and was thrown from his motorcycle; he is only responsive to pain and has an open femur fracture, but is currently protecting his airway and has no evidence of shock. We are concerned for his altered mental status, and open femur fracture, but are unable to tell if he has a spinal injury. He needs transfer for surgical management and further neurological assessment. Spinal immobilization should be maintained and he should be monitored for worsening bleeding and mental status changes.*

Case 2: A 14-year-old girl had a seizure/convulsion at school. She was brought to you by her teachers because she did not stop seizing. You administered a benzodiazepine, which caused the seizures to stop. After, you were able to perform the ABCDE survey and then a complete head-to-toe exam. She does not have a fever; she has a normal heart rate, blood pressure, and respiratory rate. She responds to voice. Her tongue is bitten and she urinated on herself; she has no other injuries or rashes.

Handover summary: *This is a 14-year-old girl who had a prolonged convulsion and was convulsing on arrival; her seizures were stopped with one 10 mg dose of diazepam and now she remains sleepy, has normal vital signs and no fever. She is being transferred for further evaluation of her seizure. Monitor the airway as she has received sedating medications (diazepam).*

Case 3: A 75-year-old man had chest pain while walking home from the market. He was brought to you by taxi. He says that the chest pain started 30 minutes ago and felt like a lot of pressure in the centre of his chest. He has no allergies. He takes a blood pressure medication, but cannot recall the medication's name. He had a heart attack 2 years ago that felt very much like the pain he was having today. His last meal was 6 hours ago. The pain started while he was walking home carrying several heavy bags, though he now has no pain. His vital signs, ABCDE survey, and head-to-toe examination are normal. You have given aspirin and started an IV line and will now handover to an inpatient provider.

Handover summary: *This is a 75-year-old man with a history of a heart attack who has had chest pain similar to his prior heart attack. The pain started while he was walking and lasted for more than 30 minutes, but is now gone. He has received aspirin and has an IV line. I am concerned he might have problems with his heart. He should be monitored for change in ABCDE or return of the chest pain.*

INTRO

ABCDE

TRAUMA

BREATHING

SHOCK

AMS

SKILLS

GLOSSARY

REFS & QUICK CARDS

Notes

GLOSSARY

ABCDE

The initial steps of any patient assessment, which includes assessing and treating **A**irway, **B**reathing, **C**irculation, **D**isability and **E**xposure.

Accessory muscle use

Use of muscles other than the diaphragm to assist in breathing (commonly the neck, chest wall, and abdominal muscles). May appear as indrawing/retractions between the ribs, or in the neck muscles.

Altered mental status (AMS)

Term used for a range of presentations from changes in behaviour or memory, to disorientation, confusion and coma.

AMS

See altered mental status.

Anaemia

Decreased concentration of red blood cells, leading to a decreased ability to carry oxygen.

Anaphylaxis

A severe allergic reaction that can cause shock.

Asthma

A condition causing mucus production and intermittent spasm in the bronchial airways, resulting in narrowing that causes wheezing.

AVPU

A system to assess level of consciousness: **A**lert, **V**erbal, **P**ain, and **U**nresponsive.

Bag-valve-mask (BVM) device

A manual handheld device consisting of an air-filled bag connected to a mask. The bag is compressed by hand to deliver a breath as the mask is held to the patient's face.

Bolus

A defined volume of fluid or other substance given rapidly, usually intravenously.

Bradycardia

Heart rate lower than normal range.

BVM

See "bag-valve-mask device".

Capillary refill

A marker of perfusion, checked by pushing on the fingernail, palms or soles and releasing to see long it takes for the colour to come back to the skin (blood flow to return). The normal range is less than 3 seconds.

Cardiopulmonary resuscitation (CPR)

Performing chest compressions and ventilation with the goal of resuscitating a patient with no pulse.

Cervical spine (C-spine)

The part of the spine in the neck, containing the first seven vertebrae.

Circumferential burn

Burns that extend around a body part can act like a rigid band and may limit blood supply (to a limb) or breathing (burn around the chest or abdomen).

Cholera

Bacterial infection causing a profound watery diarrhoea, often described as rice-water stools.

Chronic obstructive pulmonary disease (COPD)

Term describing breakdown of lung structure (emphysema) and chronic inflammation causing spasm of the lower airways and wheezing.

Coma

Prolonged state of unconsciousness.

Compartment syndrome

A condition of increased pressure from swelling in an area of the body that cannot expand, such as compartments in the forearm or lower leg. Compartment syndrome reduces blood flow to the area and may result in severe pain as well as damage to nerves and other tissues.

Confusion

Problems with clarity, recall and organization of thought.

Convulsion

See Seizure.

CPR

See cardiopulmonary resuscitation.

Crackles

High pitched sound, like crumpling of a paper bag, heard with a stethoscope. Crackles are caused by fluid in the airspaces of the lungs. Also called rales or crepitations (creps).

Crepitations

See "Crackles".

Crepitus

Crackling or popping when pressing on the skin or bones.

Cyanosis

Blue colouring to the skin or lips, resulting from low blood oxygen levels.

Decontamination

Removing a dangerous substance, such as chemicals, toxins or infectious materials, from a person's skin or clothes. Depending on the substance, this is done by brushing off the substance or irrigating with water.

Deep wound packing

Tight packing of a large or gaping wound with clean, compact gauze to ensure that external pressure can effectively compress an area of bleeding that is too large or too deep to compress otherwise.

Defibrillator

Machine that delivers high-energy electrical current to convert abnormal heart rhythms.

Dehydration

Decreased fluid in the body.

Delirium

Rapidly changing state of confusion, characterized by agitation, loss of focus and inability to interact appropriately.

Dementia

Chronic condition characterized by abnormal mental state, including loss of memory and problems with thinking. There is often no change in ability to focus on the present.

Destination planning

Planning the choice of destination facility for transport or transfer in order to best match transport time and the level of services available at the receiving facility to the patient's clinical needs.

Diabetic ketoacidosis (DKA)

A condition occurring in diabetics in which lack of insulin causes elevated blood sugar, leading to severe dehydration and build-up of acid in the blood.

Diaphoresis

Sweating.

DIB

See difficulty in breathing.

INTRO

ABCDE

TRAUMA

BREATHING

SHOCK

AMS

SKILLS

GLOSSARY

REFS & QUICK CARDS

DKA

See Diabetic Ketoacidosis.

Dilation (of blood vessels)

The enlargement or stretching of a part of the body (e.g. blood vessels).

Difficulty in breathing (DIB)

The feeling of difficulty in breathing (sometimes also called shortness of breath, or SOB) can result from many causes, including problems with the lungs, problems with oxygen, airway blockage, fast breathing, weak respiratory muscles.

Direct pressure

A way to control external bleeding (haemorrhage) from a wound by applying firm pressure with two or three fingers at the site of bleeding.

Disposition

The next step in care of a patient – this may be handover of care to another provider through admission or transfer, or discharge to home.

Drowning

Compromise of breathing from water in the lungs, usually resulting from prolonged time under water.

Eclampsia

A condition when a pregnant or newly delivered woman has seizures, high blood pressure, and protein in the urine. It can progress to coma and is life-threatening. ("Pre-eclampsia" is diagnosed based on specific criteria and identifies a woman at high-risk of progression to eclampsia.)

Ectopic pregnancy

A pregnancy outside of the uterus, most often in the fallopian tubes. As an ectopic embryo grows, it may damage the surrounding structures, causing sudden severe bleeding. Ruptured ectopic pregnancy is a surgical emergency.

Envenomation

The process by which venom is injected by the bite (or sting) of a venomous animal.

Escharotomy

A surgical procedure to cut and release burned tissue that may restrict breathing or blood supply to a limb.

Flail chest

When multiple rib fractures in more than one place cause a segment of the rib cage to be separated from the rest of the chest wall and prevent normal breathing movement.

Fluid status

The level of fluid in the body. It can be low (dehydration), normal, or high (fluid overload and/ or oedema).

Fontanelle

A gap (soft spot) between the developing bones of the skull in babies – changes in the volume of fontanelles may reflect fluid status. Fontanelles normally close between 12 and 18 months of age.

Foreign body

An object from outside the body (e.g. a foreign body in the airway).

Fracture

A broken or cracked bone.

GCS

See Glasgow Coma Scale.

Gastroenteritis

Infection or inflammation of the stomach and intestine that can cause vomiting, diarrhoea and abdominal pain.

Glasgow Coma Scale (GCS)

A system of assessing the neurologic function of a trauma patient. It is a score ranging from 3 (unresponsive) to 15 (normal) that assesses responsiveness based on eye movement, verbal response and motor response.

Guarding

Voluntary or involuntary contraction of the abdominal wall muscles when pressing on the abdomen.

Handover

A brief summary of critical patient information given by the current provider any time a patient is transferred to a new provider. Handover summarizes the clinical presentation, the care the patient has received, and alerts the new provider of any potential complications. Handover should always be given to transport providers, in addition to receiving-facility providers. Handover should also be given even when care is transferred to a new provider within the same facility.

Haemorrhage

Large volume bleeding. It may occur externally or within the body.

Haemorrhagic shock

A state of poor perfusion due to substantial blood loss.

INTRO

ABCDE

TRAUMA

BREATHING

SHOCK

AMS

SKILLS

GLOSSARY

REFS & QUICK CARDS

Haematoma

Bleeding or a collection of blood within the tissues, outside of the vascular space. Also called bruising.

Haemothorax

Blood in the space between the chest wall and the lungs.

Heart attack

(Also called myocardial infarction). Death of heart muscle due to a lack of oxygen-rich blood getting to the heart.

Heart failure

When the heart fails to pump enough blood to perfuse the organs, usually resulting in oedema in the lungs or extremities.

Hives

Multiple itchy, red and raised areas on the skin suggestive of an allergic reaction.

Human Immunodeficiency Virus (HIV)

A virus that weakens the immune system and can lead to AIDS, a syndrome of multiple infections.

Hyperthermia

High body temperature.

Hyperventilation

Increased (fast) rate of breathing.

Hyperresonance

Hollow sounds with percussion.

Hypoglycaemia

Low blood sugar.

Hypothermia

Low body temperature.

Hypotension

Blood pressure lower than the normal range.

Hypovolaemic shock

Poor perfusion due to low blood volume, which may result from decreased fluid intake or severe fluid or blood loss.

Hypoxia

Low levels of oxygen in the blood.

INTRO

ABCDE

TRAUMA

BREATHING

SHOCK

AMS

SKILLS

GLOSSARY

REFS & QUICK CARDS

Inflammation

Redness and swelling that may result from trauma, infection, allergy or other causes.

Ingestion

Swallowing a substance – generally used for dangerous substances or doses.

Inhalation injury

Inflammation or oedema of the airways or lungs resulting from breathing hot gases or irritating chemicals (most commonly smoke inhalation in the setting of fire).

Intubation

Placing a breathing tube through the mouth, down the throat, and through the vocal cords to allow ventilation of the lungs by bag device or ventilator.

Ischaemia

Inadequate oxygen and blood supply to tissues that can lead to tissue death (myocardial ischaemia, or lack of oxygen to the heart muscle, is an example).

IV (abbreviation for intravenous)

Often used to refer to an intravenous catheter, or for the intravenous route of administration of a medication or fluid.

Kangaroo care

Using skin to skin contact between a newborn infant and mother and covering the child's head and exposed body, to prevent hypothermia and promote bonding.

Laceration

A cut or slice to the tissues.

Large-bore IV

A large IV catheter is needed for rapid volume resuscitation. Ideally, these catheters should be placed in larger blood vessels (that tend to be closer to the heart, like the antecubital fossa in the arms or large veins in the neck). In adults, this is usually defined as 14- or 16-gauge, though in some settings, 18 may be the largest available gauge.

Level of consciousness

Describes the level of responsiveness or alertness to the environment.

Lethargy

Excessive drowsiness and slowness to respond.

Log roll

A method of rolling a person to the side while preventing the spine from bending. Usually performed when spinal injury is suspected to prevent additional damage.

Nasal flaring

The widening of nostrils during breathing – it results from increased effort, and is a sign of difficulty in breathing.

Nasopharyngeal airway (NPA)

A rubber tube inserted through the nostril that reaches to the opening of the throat to allow air to pass.

Needle decompression

Insertion of a needle into the chest wall to relieve the pressure of a tension pneumothorax.

Oedema

Abnormal swelling or fluid build-up in the body tissues, outside the vascular space.

Oral rehydration solution (ORS)

A water, glucose, and salt mixture given by mouth or nasogastric tube to dehydrated patients to replace fluid losses.

Orientation

Describes a person's relationship to the surrounding world, including the ability to accurately identify one's own name and location, as well as the current time and date.

Oropharyngeal airway (OPA)

A plastic device inserted through the mouth that reaches to the opening of the throat to prevent the tongue from blocking the airway and allows air to pass.

ORS

See "Oral rehydration solution".

Oxygen (O2) saturation

Percent of oxygen in the blood.

Parkland Formula

A formula used to estimate the amount of IV fluid needed for resuscitation of a burn patient over the first 24 hours after the burn. It is: 4 ml fluid X weight in kilograms X total burn surface area. Half should be given over the first 8 hours, and half over the next 16 hours.

Percussion

Tapping on the chest wall to assess the lungs. The quality of the sound on tapping may indicate fluid or air in the lungs.

Perfusion

The delivery of blood to body tissues.

Pericardial effusion

Fluid in the sac around the heart (the pericardium).

Pericardial tamponade

A critical build-up of fluid in the sac around the heart (the pericardium) that compresses the heart and interferes with normal pumping of blood to the body, leading to shock.

Personal protective equipment (PPE)

Equipment meant to be worn by a person to protect from infection or injury. This can include gloves, goggles, and protective clothing such as aprons or fluid resistant gowns.

Pleural effusion

Abnormal fluid collection around the lung that can cause difficulty in breathing and even lung collapse. Common causes include tuberculosis and other infections, heart failure and cancer.

Pleuritic pain

Pain that is worse with breathing, usually caused by inflammation.

Pneumonia

Infection of the lungs.

Pneumothorax

Air in the space between the lungs and the chest wall (pleural space) that causes the lung to collapse.

Pre-eclampsia

See Eclampsia.

Priapism

Persistent, abnormal erection of the penis.

Psychosis

Broadly defined as loss of contact with reality.

Pulmonary embolism

Blood clot travelling to and blocking the vessels of the lungs. The most common source is the legs.

Pulse oximeter

Device that detects oxygen saturation (the percentage of red blood cells saturated with oxygen).

Rabies

A virus that is transmitted through animal bites that affects the brain and nerves and can cause altered mental status.

Rebound tenderness

Pain that occurs when releasing pressure on the abdomen (as opposed to when pressing on the abdomen).

INTRO

ABCDE

TRAUMA

BREATHING

SHOCK

AMS

SKILLS

GLOSSARY

REFS & QUICK CARDS

Resuscitation

Time-sensitive interventions performed in an attempt to manage life-threatening conditions.

Retractions (sometimes also called "in-drawing" or "recessions")

The visible pulling in of tissues between the ribs or around the collarbones with strained inspiration. Retractions are a sign of serious difficulty in breathing.

SAMPLE history

An approach to asking key history findings for all patients. SAMPLE stands for: S – Signs and Symptoms, A – Allergies, M – Medications, P – Past history, L – Last oral intake, E – Events surrounding the illness or injury.

Seizure

Also called convulsions or fits. Abnormal electrical activity in the brain, often seen as altered mental status with abnormal repetitive movements. Seizures may be a primary condition or may be caused by infection, injury, toxins or chemical balance problems.

Shock

A state where organs do not get enough blood and oxygen (poor perfusion), leading to organs not working properly.

Skin pinch testing

An easy way to check hydration status in children by pinching the skin, usually on the abdomen. Well-hydrated skin should return to normal in less than 2 seconds.

Sprain

A stretched, pulled, or torn ligament.

Stridor

A high pitched sound on breathing in that is caused by swelling or a physical obstruction of the upper airway.

Stroke

Death of brain tissue due to ischaemia from either blood clot or haemorrhage.

Sucking chest wound

A wound in the chest wall that allows air in and out of the chest cavity, indicating an open pneumothorax.

Tachycardia

Heart rate faster than normal range.

Tachypnoea

Rapid breathing.

Tension pneumothorax

Occurs when a pneumothorax causes sufficient pressure inside the chest cavity that blood vessels collapse (reducing the amount of blood that can return to the heart, and the heart cannot fill or pump enough blood to maintain perfusion of the organs).

Tracheal shift

Describes a change in the position of the trachea to either side of midline, a finding sometimes associated with tension pneumothorax.

Trauma primary survey

The trauma primary survey is another term for the ABCDE approach in injured patients. It includes initial assessment of an injured person and management of all immediately life-threatening injuries, in order of priority. The primary survey consists of the ABCDE: Airway, Breathing, Circulation, Disability and Exposure.

Trauma secondary survey

The head-to-toe (front and back) examination of the trauma patient that includes taking a SAMPLE history. The purpose of this survey is to identify and treat all injuries, with priority given to any hidden life-threatening conditions that were missed by the primary survey.

Tripod position

Sitting upright with neck extended but leaning slightly forward with hands on knees. People with severe difficulty in breathing will often sit in this position.

Wheezing

A whistling sound made when breathing out due to inflammation in the lungs, suggestive of lower airway swelling.

WHO sources

Emergency Triage Assessment and Treatment (ETAT). Geneva: World Health Organization; 2005. June 2016 update.

Integrated Management of Adolescent and Adult Illness (IMAI) District Clinician Manual. Volume 1 and 2. Geneva: World Health Organization; 2011:Chapter 2–4; 6–8.

Pocket book for hospital care of children. Second edition. Geneva: World Health Organization; 2013.

Basic Emergency Care
Quick Cards

INTRO

ABCDE

TRAUMA

BREATHING

SHOCK

AMS

SKILLS

GLOSSARY

REFS & QUICK CARDS

ABCDE APPROACH

REMEMBER... Always check for signs of trauma [see also TRAUMA card]

		ASSESSMENT FINDINGS	IMMEDIATE MANAGEMENT
Airway	A	Unconscious with limited or no air movement	If **NO TRAUMA**: head-tilt and chin-lift, use OPA or NPA to keep airway open, place in recovery position or position of comfort. If possible **TRAUMA**: use jaw thrust with c-spine protection and place OPA to keep the airway open (no NPA if facial trauma).
		Foreign body in airway	Remove visible foreign body. Encourage coughing. • If **unable** to cough: chest/abdominal thrusts/back blows as indicated • If patient becomes unconscious: CPR
		Gurgling	Open airway as above, suction (avoid gagging).
		Stridor	Keep patient calm and allow position of comfort. • For signs of anaphylaxis: give IM adrenaline • For hypoxia: give oxygen
Breathing	B	Signs of abnormal breathing or hypoxia	Give oxygen. Assist ventilation with BVM if breathing NOT adequate.
		Wheeze	Give salbutamol. For signs of anaphylaxis: give IM adrenaline.
		Signs of tension pneumothorax (absent sounds / hyperresonance on one side WITH hypotension, distended neck veins)	Perform needle decompression, give oxygen and IV fluids. Will need chest tube
		Signs of opiate overdose (AMS and slow breathing with small pupils)	Give naloxone.
Circulation	C	Signs of poor perfusion/shock	If **no pulse**, follow relevant CPR protocols. Give oxygen and IV fluids.
		Signs of internal or external bleeding	Control external bleeding. Give IV fluids.
		Signs of pericardial tamponade (poor perfusion with distended neck veins and muffled heart sounds)	Give IV fluids, oxygen. Will need rapid pericardial drainage
Disability	D	Altered mental status (AMS)	If NO TRAUMA, place in recovery position.
		Seizure	Give benzodiazepine.
		Seizure in pregnancy (or after recent delivery)	Give magnesium sulphate.
		Hypoglycaemia	Give glucose if <3.5 mmol/L or unknown.
		Signs of opiate overdose (AMS with slow breathing with small pupils)	Give naloxone.
		Signs of life-threatening brain mass or bleed (AMS with unequal pupils)	Raise head of bed, monitor airway. Will need rapid transfer for neurosurgical services
Exposure	E	Remove wet clothing and dry skin thoroughly.	
		Remove jewelry, watches and constrictive clothing	
		Prevent hypothermia and protect modesty.	
		Snake bite	Immobilize extremity. Send picture of snake with patient. Call for anti-venom if relevant.

If cause unknown, remember trauma: Examine the entire body and always consider hidden injuries [see also TRAUMA card]

REMEMBER: PATIENTS WITH ABNORMAL ABCDE FINDINGS MAY NEED RAPID HANDOVER/TRANSFER. PLAN EARLY.

Pulse rate: 60–100 beats per minute
Respiratory rate: 10–20 breaths per minute
Systolic blood pressure >90 mmHg
Oxygen Saturation > 92%

Estimating systolic blood pressure
(not reliable in children and the elderly):
Carotid (neck) pulse → SBP ≥ 60 mmHg
Femoral (groin) pulse → SBP ≥ 70 mmHg
Radial (wrist) pulse → SBP ≥80 mmHg

SAMPLE History

Signs & Symptoms
Allergies
Medications
PMH
Last oral intake
Events

SPECIAL CONSIDERATIONS IN THE ASSESSMENT OF CHILDREN

A
- Children have bigger heads and tongues, and shorter, softer necks than adults. Position airway as appropriate for age.
- Always consider foreign bodies.

B
- Look for signs of increased work of breathing (e.g. chest indrawing, retractions, nasal flaring).
- Listen for abnormal breath sounds (e.g. grunting, stridor, or silent chest).

AGE	RESPIRATORY RATE (breaths per minute)
<2 months	40–60
2–12 months	25–50
1–5 years	20–40

C
- Signs of poor perfusion in children include: slow capillary refill, decreased urine output, lethargy, sunken fontanelle, poor skin pinch
- Look for signs of anaemia and malnourishment (adjust fluids).
- Remember that children may not always report trauma and may have serious internal injury with few external signs.

AGE (in years)	NORMAL HEART RATE (beats per minute)
<1	100–160
1–3	90–150
4–5	80–140

D
- Always check AVPU
- Hypoglycaemia is common in ill children.
- Check for tone and response to stimulus.
- Look for lethargy or irritability.

E
INFANTS AND CHILDREN HAVE DIFFICULTY MAINTAINING TEMPERATURE
- Remove wet clothing and dry skin thoroughly. Place infants skin-to-skin when possible.
- For hypothermia, cover the head (but be sure mouth and nose are clear).
- For hyperthermia, unbundle tightly wrapped babies.

DANGER SIGNS IN CHILDREN

- Signs of airway obstruction (unable to swallow saliva/drooling or stridor)
- Increased breathing effort (fast breathing, nasal flaring, grunting, chest indrawing or retractions)
- Cyanosis (blue colour of the skin, especially at the lips and fingertips)
- Altered mental status (including lethargy or unusual sleepiness, confusion, disorientation)
- Moves only when stimulated or no movement at all (AVPU other than "A")
- Not feeding well, cannot drink or breastfeed or vomiting everything
- Seizures/convulsions
- Low body temperature (hypothermia)

ESTIMATED WEIGHT in KILOGRAMS for CHILDREN 1–10 YEARS OLD:
[age in years + 4] x 2

APPROACH TO THE PATIENT WITH TRAUMA

Key findings from the Trauma Primary Survey [see also ABCDE card]

	ASSESSMENT FINDINGS	IMMEDIATE MANAGEMENT
Airway A	Not speaking, with limited or no air movement	Use jaw thrust with c-spine protection. Suction if needed, remove visible foreign objects. Place OPA to keep the airway open.
	Signs of possible airway injury (neck haematoma or wound, crepitus, stridor)	Give oxygen. Monitor closely-- swelling can rapidly block the airway. → Will need advanced airway management
	Signs of possible airway burns (soot around the mouth or nose, burned facial hair, facial burns)	Give oxygen. Monitor closely-- swelling can rapidly close the airway. → Will need advanced airway management
Breathing B	Signs of tension pneumothorax (hypotension with absent breath sounds/hyperresonance on one side, distended neck veins)	Perform needle decompression. Give oxygen, IV fluids. → Will need chest tube
	Open (sucking) chest wound	Give oxygen, place 3-sided dressing, monitor for tension pneumothorax. → Will need chest tube
	Breathing not adequate	Give oxygen, assist ventilation with BVM.
	Large burns of chest or abdomen (or circumferential burn to limb)	Give IV fluids per burn size, give oxygen, remove constricting clothing/jewelry. → May need escharotomy
	Signs of flail chest (section of chest wall moving in opposite direction with breathing)	Give oxygen. → May need advanced airway management and assisted ventilation
	Signs of haemothorax (decreased breath sounds on one side, dull sounds with percussion)	Give oxygen, IV fluids. → Will need chest tube
Circulation C	Signs of shock (capillary refill >3 sec, hypotension, tachycardia)	Give oxygen, IV fluids, control external bleeding, splint femur/pelvis as indicated.
	Uncontrolled external bleeding	Apply pressure, deep wound packing or tourniquet as indicated.
	Signs of tamponade (poor perfusion, distended neck veins, muffled heart sounds)	Give IV fluids, oxygen.
Disability D	Signs of brain injury (AMS with wound, deformity or bruising of head/face)	Immobilize cervical spine, check glucose, give nothing by mouth. → Will need neurosurgical care
	Signs of open skull fracture (as above, with blood or fluid from the ears/nose)	As above, and give IV antibiotics per local protocol.

REMEMBER: INJURED PATIENTS WITH ABNORMAL ABCDE FINDINGS MAY NEED RAPID HANDOVER/TRANSFER TO A SURGICAL SERVICE. PLAN EARLY.

MANAGEMENT OF SPECIFIC CONDITIONS

Facial fracture	Immobilize cervical spine if indicated, give IV antibiotics for open fractures, avoid nasal airway/ nasogastric tubes.
Penetrating eye injury	Avoid pressure on the eye, stabilize but do not remove foreign objects, give antibiotics and tetanus, elevate head of bed.
Open abdominal wound	Give IV fluids, nothing by mouth. Cover visible bowel with sterile gauze soaked in sterile saline, give antibiotics.
Pelvic fracture	Give IV fluids, stabilize with sheet or pelvic binder.
Fracture with poor limb perfusion	Reduce fracture, splint.
Open fracture	Irrigate well, dress wound, splint, give antibiotics, rapid handover for operative management.
Penetrating object	Leave object in place and stabilize it to prevent further injury.
Crush injury	Give IV fluids, monitor urine output, monitor for compartment syndrome.
Burn injury	Assess size and calculate fluid needs, give IV fluids and oxygen, monitor for airway oedema.
Blast injury	Give oxygen, treat burns as below, give IV fluids, monitor closely for delayed effects of internal injury.

REMEMBER: INJURED PATIENTS WITH WOUNDS, INCLUDING BURNS AND OPEN FRACTURES, NEED TETANUS VACCINATION.

HIGH-RISK MECHANISMS AND INJURIES

High-Risk Mechanisms	High-Risk Injuries
• Pedestrian or cyclist hit by a vehicle • Motorcycle crash or any vehicle crash with unrestrained occupants • Falls from heights greater than 3 metres (or twice a child's height) • Gunshot or stabbing • Explosion or fire in an enclosed space.	• Penetrating injuries to head, neck or torso • Blast or crush injuries • Flail chest • Two or more large bone fractures, or pelvic fracture • Spinal injury • Limb paralysis • Amputation above wrist or ankle

SPECIAL CONSIDERATIONS IN CHILDREN

• Children can look well but then deteriorate quickly.

• Children have more flexible bones than adults and can have serious internal injuries with few external signs.

• Use caution when calculating fluid and medication dosages. Use exact weight whenever possible.

• Watch carefully for hypothermia and hypoglycaemia.

DISPOSITION

Conditions that require handover or transfer to a specialist unit include:

• ABCDE finding that has required intervention	• Altered mental status
• Evidence of internal bleeding	• Trauma during pregnancy
• Any pneumothorax or sucking chest wound	• ABCDE abnormalities or any chest /abdomen injury in a child
• Shock, even if treated successfully	• Significant burn injuries

Considerations for transfer:

• Any patient who has required oxygen should have oxygen during transport and after handover.
• For signs of shock, ensure IV fluid started and continued during transfer.
• Control any external bleeding and monitor site closely during transport.

APPROACH TO THE PATIENT WITH DIFFICULTY IN BREATHING

Key ABCDE Findings (Always perform a complete ABCDE approach first!)

IF YOU FIND...	REMEMBER...
Choking, coughing	Foreign body
Stridor	Partial airway obstruction due to foreign body or inflammation (from infection, chemical exposure or burn)
Facial swelling	Severe allergic reaction, medication effect
Drooling	Indicates a blockage to swallowing
Soot around the mouth or nose, burned facial hair, facial burns	Smoke inhalation and airway burns – rapid swelling can block the airway
Signs of chest wall trauma	Rib fracture, flail chest, pneumothorax, contusion, tamponade
Decreased breath sounds on one side	Pneumothorax (consider tension pneumothorax if with hypotension and hyperresonance to percussion), haemothorax, large pleural effusion/pneumonia
Decreased breath sounds and crackles on both sides	Pulmonary oedema, heart failure
Wheezing	Asthma, allergic reaction, COPD
Fast or deep breathing	DKA
Low blood pressure, tachycardia, muffled heart sounds	Pericardial tamponade
Altered mental status with small pupils and slow breathing	Opioid overdose

Key Findings from the SAMPLE History and Secondary Exam

IF YOU FIND...	REMEMBER...
DIB worse with exertion or activity	Heart failure, heart attack
DIB that began with choking or during eating	Foreign body, allergic reaction
History of fever, cough	Pneumonia, infection
Pesticide exposure	Poisoning
Recent fall or other trauma	Rib fracture, flail chest, pneumothorax, contusion, tamponade
Known allergies, allergen exposure, bite or sting	Allergic reaction
Recent medication or dose change	Allergic reaction or side effect
History of opioid or sedative drug use	Overdose
History of wheezing	Asthma or COPD
History of diabetes	DKA
History of tuberculosis or malignancy	Pericardial tamponade, pleural effusion
History of heart failure	Pulmonary oedema
History of sickle cell disease	Acute chest syndrome

CRITICAL ACTIONS FOR HIGH-RISK CONDITIONS

CHOKING	STRIDOR	WHEEZING	SEVERE INFECTION	TRAUMA
unable to cough, not making sounds	*high pitched sounds on breathing IN*	*high pitched sounds on breathing OUT*		
Remove any visible foreign body	Keep patient calm and allow position of comfort	Give salbutamol	Oxygen	Oxygen
Perform age-appropriate chest/abdominal thrusts or back blows	IM adrenaline for suspected allergic reaction	IM adrenaline for suspected allergic reaction	Antibiotics	Needle decompression and IV fluids for tension pneumothorax
CPR if becomes unconscious	Oxygen if concern for hypoxia	Oxygen if concern for hypoxia	Oral/IV fluids as appropriate	Three-sided dressing for sucking chest wound
	Early handover/transfer for advanced airway management			Rapid transfer to surgical service

SPECIAL CONSIDERATIONS IN CHILDREN

THE FOLLOWING ARE DANGER SIGNS IN CHILDREN WITH BREATHING COMPLAINTS:

- Fast breathing
- Increased breathing effort (chest indrawing/retractions)
- Cyanosis
- Altered mental status (including lethargy)

- Poor feeding or drinking, or vomits everything
- Seizures/convulsions, current or recent
- Drooling or stridor when calm
- Hypothermia

Wheezing in children is often caused by an object inhaled into the airway, viral infection or asthma.

Stridor in children is often caused by an object stuck in the airway or airway swelling from infection.

Fast or deep breathing can indicate diabetic crisis (DKA), which may be the first sign of diabetes in a child.

FAST BREATHING MAY BE THE ONLY SIGN OF A SERIOUS BREATHING PROBLEM IN A CHILD.

DISPOSITION

Salbutamol and IM adrenaline effects last for about 3 hours, and life-threatening symptoms may recur. Monitor closely, always have repeat dose available during transport and caution new providers at handover.

Naloxone lasts approximately 1 hour, and most opioids last longer. Monitor closely, always have repeat dose available during transport and caution new providers.

Following immersion in water (drowning), a person may develop delayed breathing problems after several hours. Monitor closely and caution new providers.

Never leave patients with difficulty in breathing unmonitored during handover/transfer.

Make transfer arrangements as early as possible for any patient who may require intubation or assisted ventilation.

APPROACH TO THE PATIENT WITH SHOCK

Key ABCDE Findings (Always perform a complete ABCDE approach first!)

IF YOU FIND...	REMEMBER...
Difficulty breathing, stridor/wheezing, skin rash, swelling of mouth	Severe allergic reaction
Hypotension with absent breath sounds and hyperresonance on one side, distended neck veins	Tension pneumothorax
Distended neck veins, muffled heart sounds, tachycardia, hypotension	Pericardial tamponade
Sweet smelling breath, deep or rapid breathing	DKA
History of trauma or no known cause	Hidden sources of significant blood loss (stomach, intestines, intra-abdominal, chest, long-bone trauma) or spinal injury

Key Findings from the SAMPLE History and Secondary Exam

IF YOU FIND...	REMEMBER...
Vomiting and diarrhoea	Ask about contacts and report cases per protocol.
Black or bloody vomit or stool	Stomach or intestinal bleeding
Rapid or deep breathing, dehydration, high glucose, sweet-smelling breath, history of frequent urination or known diabetes	Diabetic ketoacidosis
Burns	Severe fluid loss (calculate fluid needs based on burn size)
Fever or HIV	Infection
Recent fall or other trauma	Internal AND external bleeding
Pale conjunctiva or malnutrition	Severe anemia (adjust fluids)
Chest pain	Heart attack (give aspirin if indicated)
Vaginal bleeding	Pregnancy and non-pregnancy related bleeding
Numbness, weakness or shock that does not improve with fluids	Spinal shock (immobilize spine if indicated)

CRITICAL ACTIONS FOR HIGH-RISK CONDITIONS

For all shock:

- **Give oxygen**
- **Give IV fluids**
  - ADULTS: 1 liter RL or NS bolus
  - CHILDREN with NO severe anaemia, NO malnutrition, NO fluid overload: 10–20 ml/kg bolus
  - CHILDREN with malnutrition or severe anaemia: give 10–15 ml/kg dextrose-containing fluid **over 1 hour** and assess for fluid overload every 5 minutes.
  - For suspected heart attack with shock, give smaller boluses, and monitor closely for fluid overload.
- **Monitor vital signs, mental status, breathing and urine output**

AND for specific conditions:

SEVERE ALLER-GIC REACTION	TENSION PNEUMO-THORAX	TAMPONADE	FEVER	WATERY DIARRHOEA	POSTPARTUM BLEEDING	DKA	TRAUMA
IM adrenaline Monitor for recurrence, may need repeat doses	Rapid needle decompression Transfer for chest tube	Rapid transfer to advanced provider for drainage	Antibiotics (and anti-malarials if indicated) Assess for source of infection	Full contact precautions Monitor output and continue fluids Assess for cholera and notify public health authorities	Oxytocin and uterine massage Direct pressure for perineal and vaginal tears Rapid transfer to advanced obstetric care	Close monitoring for fluid overload in children Handover/transfer for insulin	Control external haemorrhage with direct pressure, wound packing, tourniquet if indicated Calculate fluid needs based on burn size Rapid transfer for surgery/transfusion as needed

SPECIAL CONSIDERATIONS IN CHILDREN

ASSESSING SHOCK IN CHILDREN

The 2016 WHO guidelines for the care of critically ill children use the presence of three clinical features to define shock:

- Cold extremities
- Weak and fast pulse
- Capillary refill greater than 3 seconds

Additional important considerations include:

- Young children may not be able to drink enough fluid on their own.
- Children have larger surface area to volume ratio and can lose fluids more quickly than adults.
- For a child in shock WITH severe malnutrition or fluid overload, add dextrose and reduce fluids to 10–15 ml/kg over 1 hour.

In children *without* severe malnutrition, severe anaemia or fluid overload, give fluid resuscitation over 30 minutes.

WEIGHT (kg)	FLUID VOLUME (15ml/kg)
4	60
6	90
10	150
14	210
20	300
30	450

Other important signs of poor perfusion include:

- Sunken eyes; sunken fontanelles in infants
- Abnormal skin pinch test
- Pallor (dehydration with anaemia is more difficult to treat)
- Decreased and dark urine (number of nappies for infants)
- Low blood pressure
- Fast breathing
- Altered mental status
- Very dry mouth and lips
- Lethargy (excessive drowsiness, slow to respond, not interactive)

DISPOSITION

Patients with shock should be at a unit capable of providing IV fluid resuscitation, blood transfusion, and/or surgery, depending on the type of shock.

Maintain fluids during transport. Repeat ABCDE approach and monitor perfusion and breathing closely at all times.

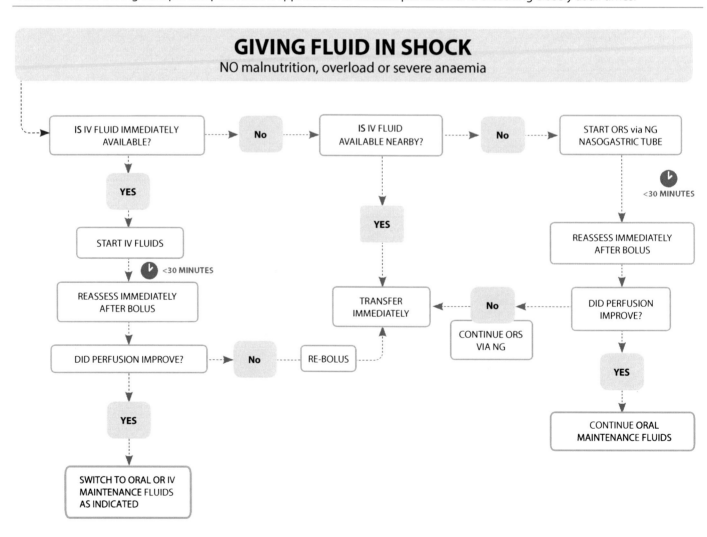

GIVING FLUID IN SHOCK
NO malnutrition, overload or severe anaemia

APPROACH TO THE PATIENT WITH ALTERED MENTAL STATUS (AMS)

Key ABCDE Findings (Always perform a complete ABCDE approach first!)

IF YOU FIND...	REMEMBER...
Tachypnoea	Hypoxia, DKA, toxic ingestion
Poor perfusion/shock	Infection, internal bleeding
Tachycardia with normal perfusion	Alcohol withdrawal
Coma	Hypoxia, high or low blood glucose, DKA and toxic ingestion
Hypoglycaemia	Infection, medication side effect (eg, diabetes medications, quinine)
Very small pupils with slow breathing	Opioid overdose
Seizure/convulsion	Abnormal glucose, infection, toxic ingestion (eg, TB meds) or withdrawal (eg, alcohol). Consider eclampsia if current pregnancy or recent delivery.
Weakness on one side or unequal pupil size	Brain mass or bleed
Signs of trauma or unknown cause of AMS	Consider brain injury (with possible spine injury)

Key Findings from SAMPLE History and Secondary Exam

IF YOU FIND...	REMEMBER...
History of wheezing	Severe COPD crisis can cause AMS
History of diabetes	High or low blood sugar, DKA
History of epilepsy	Post-seizure confusion and sleepiness should improve over minutes to hours. Prolonged AMS or multiple convulsions without waking up in between require further workup.
History of agricultural work or known pesticide exposure	Organophosphate poisoning
History of regular alcohol use	Alcohol withdrawal
History of substance use or depression	Acute intoxication, accidental or intentional overdose
History of HIV	Infection, medication side effect
Rash on the lower abdomen or legs or bulging fontanelle in infants	Brain infection (meningitis)
Fever/Hyperthermia	Infectious, toxic, and environmental causes

CRITICAL ACTIONS FOR HIGH-RISK CONDITIONS
(Always check blood glucose in AMS, or give glucose if unable to check.)

HYPOGLYCAEMIA	OPIOID OVERDOSE	LIFE-THREATENING INFECTIONS	SEVERE DEHYDRATION	TOXIC EXPOSURE OR WITHDRAWAL
Give glucose	Naloxone	IV fluids	IV fluids	Gather history and consult advanced provider for locally-appropriate antidotes.
Evaluate for infection	Monitor need for repeat doses (many opioids last longer than naloxone)	Antibiotics	Assess for infection	
Monitor for return of hypoglycaemia		For AMS with fever or rash, consider brain infection (meningitis) – isolate patient and wear mask.	Consider DKA	Treat alcohol withdrawal with benzodiazepine.
		Cool if indicated for very high fever (avoid shivering).		Decontaminate for chemical exposures (eg, pesticides).

PAEDIATRIC CONSIDERATIONS

ALWAYS consider unwitnessed toxic ingestion	Ask about any medications in the household, and any chemicals (eg cleaning products, antifreeze) in or near the house.
Check and regularly re-check blood glucose	Low blood glucose is common in ill young children. High blood glucose can present with AMS and dehydration.
AVOID hypothermia	Keep skin-to-skin with mother, cover child's head. Uncover only the parts you need to see, one at a time, during exam.
Danger signs with ingestions • Stridor • Oral chemical burns	Monitor closely and arrange handover/transfer for advanced airway management.
Monitor fluid status closely	Paediatric patients are more susceptible to both fluid losses and fluid overload.

DISPOSITION CONSIDERATIONS

Patients with AMS who may not be able to protect the airway should never be left alone. Monitor closely and give direct handover to new provider.

Naloxone lasts approximately 1 hour. Most opioids last longer-- always alert new providers that patients may need repeat doses.

Hypoglycaemia often recurs. Alert new providers to monitor blood glucose frequently in any patient who has been treated for hypoglycaemia.

MEDICATIONS

MEDICATION	DOSAGE	INDICATION
Adrenaline (Epinephrine)	**Solution: 1mg in 1ml ampoule (1:1000)** **Adults:** 50 kg or above: 0.5 mg **IM** (0.5 ml of 1:1000) 40 kg: 0.4 mg (0.4 ml **IM** of 1:1000) 30 kg: 0.3 mg (0.3 ml **IM** of 1:1000) Repeat every 5 minutes as needed **Children:** <u>Anaphylaxis</u>: 0.15 mg **IM** (0.15ml of 1:1000). Repeat every 5–15 minutes as needed <u>Severe Asthma</u>: 0.01 mg/kg **IM** up to 0.3mg. Repeat every 15 minutes as needed	Anaphylaxis/severe allergic reaction and severe wheezing
Acetylsalicylic acid (Aspirin)	**Oral Tablet: 100 mg, 300 mg** 300 mg (preferably chewed or in water) immediately as single dose.	Suspected heart attack
Diazepam	**Oral Tablet: 2 mg, 5 mg** **Solution: 5 mg /1 ml ampoule** **Adults:** First dose: 10 mg slow IV push or 20 mg rectally Second dose after 10 minutes: 5 mg slow IV push or 10 mg rectally Maximum IV Dose: 30 mg **Children:** First dose: 0.2 mg/kg slow IV push or 0.5 mg/kg rectally. Can repeat half of first dose after 10 minutes if seizures/convulsions continue. Max IV Dose: 20 mg **MONITOR BREATHING CLOSELY in all patients given diazepam.**	Seizures/ convulsions
Glucose (Dextrose)	**Solution: 50% dextrose (D50), 25% dextrose (D25), or 10% Dextrose (D10)** **Adults and children greater than 40kg:** 25–50 ml **IV** of D50, or 125–250 ml **IV** of D10 **Children up to 40kg:** 5 ml/kg **IV** of D10 (PREFERRED) 2 ml/kg **IV** of D25 1 ml/kg **IV** of D50 **If no IV access:** 2–5 ml of 50% Dextrose **OR** sugar solution in buccal space	Hypoglycaemia (low blood sugar)
Magnesium Sulphate	**Solution: 1 g in 2 ml ampoule (50% or 500 mg/ml), 5 g in 10 ml ampoule (50% or 500 mg/ml)** Give 4 g **IV** (dilute to a 20% solution and give 20ml) <u>**slowly**</u> over 20 minutes **AND** give 10 g **IM:** 5 g (10 ml of 50% solution) with 1 ml of 2% lidocaine **in each buttock.** **If unable to give IV, give 10 g IM injection only (as above, 5 g in each buttock).** **If seizures/convulsions recur:** after 15 minutes give additional 2 g (10 ml of 20%) **IV** over 20 minutes. **If transport delayed continue:** Give 5 g of 50% solution **IM** with 1 ml of 2% lidocaine every 4h in alternate buttocks.	Eclampsia or Pregnant with seizure/convulsion
Naloxone	**Solution: 400 mcg/ml (hydrochloride) in 1 ml ampoule** **IV:** 100 mcg single dose **OR** **IM:** 400 mcg single dose May repeat every 5 minutes as needed. May require 0.4 mg/hr infusion for several hours for long-acting opioids.	Opioid overdose

MEDICATION	DOSAGE	INDICATION
Oxytocin	**Solution: 10 IU in 1ml ampule** **Initial Dose:** Give 10 IU IM **AND** start IV fluids with 20 IU/L at 60 drops/minute. **Once placenta is delivered, continue** IV fluids with 20 IU/L at 30 drops/minute if still bleeding. **If placenta has to be manually removed or uterus does not contract:** Repeat 10 IU IM. **Continue** IV fluids with 20 IU/L at 20 drops/minute for one hour after bleeding stops. **Max Dose:** 3 L of IV fluids containing oxytocin.	Treatment of postpartum haemorrhage
Paracetamol (acetaminophen)	**Oral Tablet: 250 mg, 500 mg.** **Rectal Suppositories: 250 mg, 500 mg** **Adults:** 500 mg–1 g oral/rectal every 6hrs Max 4 g daily or max 2 g daily if liver impairment, cirrhosis **Children:** 10–15 mg/kg oral/rectal up to six times per day	Mild to moderate pain, fever, headache
Salbutamol (Albuterol)	**Inhaler: 100 mcg per puff** • **Adult:** Prime with 5 puffs and give 2 puffs via spacer every 2 minutes until improved. • **Child:** Prime with 5 puffs and give 2 puffs into spacer. Keep spacer in mouth for 3–5 breaths. Repeat until 6 puffs given for < 5 years, or 12 puffs for > 5 years. **Nebulizer: (ADULT)** 5 mg in 5 ml sterile saline. **(CHILD)** 2.5 mg in 3 ml sterile saline. *For severe wheezing, above doses can be given several times in an hour.*	Severe wheezing
Tetanus Vaccine	**IM Injection: 0.5 ml** (Give for children not up to date; adults with none in 5 years; or status unknown)	Wounds (including burns and open fractures)

TRANSFER AND HANDOVER

Arrange transfer

- Check that patient needs match the available services at the destination facility (eg, operating theatre open, blood available)
- Communicate directly with an accepting provider at the receiving facility prior to departure
- Ensure that destination facility can be reached in time given patient condition
- Ensure that patient and family are aware of reasons, plan, and destination for transport
- Record family contact name and number in sending facility chart and in paperwork sent with patient
- Secure patient valuables for transport (whenever possible, leave with family)
- A brief written record (including name, date of birth, clinical presentation and all interventions) should ALWAYS accompany the patient.

Prepare for needs during transport

- PPE for staff
- Airway equipment and suction (check if working before departure)
- Adequate oxygen (with replacement tank if needed) and bag valve mask (BVM)
- IV access: Check that IV is secured prior to transport; consider second IV or backup supply
- Medications: Bring additional doses of medications and fluids, and consider other medications that may be needed
- Prepare for new or recurrent symptoms.
- Seizure/convulsion patients: place pads/pillows around patient to limit injury from a seizure during transport.
- Watch for vomiting and ensure that airway remains clear, particularly for those with cervical spine immobilization.
- Check that there is adequate fuel for transport.
- Ensure that telephone or radio is present in vehicle and working

Patient positioning

- Position patient for best airway opening and breathing.
- Use recovery position if no trauma.
- If >20 weeks pregnant and NO spine injury: Place pillows along the length of her right back to tilt patient onto her left side. This avoids compression of the large blood vessels by the pregnant uterus.
- Check that cervical spine has been immobilized if indicated.
- Possible spine injury: use backboard and log-roll manoeuvre to move patients. Check for pressure spots every 2 hours; pad areas with soft material as needed. If >20-weeks pregnant: Tip backboard slightly to the left using a wedge or other materials.
- Splint or immobilize fractures to protect soft tissues and decrease pain and bleeding.

On-going care during transport

- Re-assess the ABCDE approach at least every 15 minutes, including repeat vital signs and glucose checks if patient has been hypoglycaemic
- Control bleeding prior to transport and monitor site for new bleeding
- Perform regular re-assessment of any splinted extremity
- Continue necessary treatments (e.g. oxygen, IV fluids, oxytocin, glucose)
- Keep the patient from getting too hot or too cold during transport.

Paediatric Considerations

- Prepare appropriate size equipment and weight-adjusted dosages of critical medications.
- Bring a family member or friend, and tell the receiving facility who is accompanying the child.
- Remember that critically ill or injured children can look well initially and then worsen quickly. Monitor closely.
- Hypothermia and hypoglycaemia are common in children. Monitor closely.

SBAR handover

- **S**ituation: Basic patient information (e.g. age, sex); chief complaint (the patient's initial description of the problem, such as difficulty in breathing for 3 days, or arm pain after a fall)
- **B**ackground: 2–4 most important and relevant aspects of patient's case and/or condition; important ABCDE findings/interventions.
- **A**ssessment: What you think is wrong with the patient; reason for the handover/transfer.
- **R**ecommendations: next steps in treatment plan; potential worsening of the patient's condition (e.g. need for close airway observation if inhalation burn is suspected); cautions regarding prior therapies or interventions (e.g. time of last adrenaline dose to anticipate return symptoms, need to monitor mental status if sedating medications have been given, need to monitor 3-way dressing for clotting, etc.).